TOBACCO & YOUR HEALTH:
THE SMOKING CONTROVERSY

McGRAW-HILL
SERIES IN
HEALTH EDUCATION

Deobold B. Van Dalen, *Consulting Editor*

Cohen THE DRUG DILEMMA

Diehl TOBACCO AND YOUR HEALTH:
THE SMOKING CONTROVERSY

Dalrymple SEX IS FOR REAL:
HUMAN SEXUALITY AND
SEXUAL RESPONSIBILITY

TOBACCO &
YOUR HEALTH:
THE SMOKING
CONTROVERSY

HAROLD S. DIEHL, M.D.
Emeritus Professor of Public Health and
Dean of the Medical Sciences, University of Minnesota
Special Consultant for Research and Medical Affairs
American Cancer Society

HV
5733
D5

McGraw-Hill Book Company
New York   St. Louis   San Francisco   London
Sydney   Toronto   Mexico   Panama

TOBACCO &
YOUR HEALTH:
THE SMOKING
CONTROVERSY

07-016875-X
07-016876-8

Library of Congress Catalog Card Number 69-13216

67890 VBVB 765432

To my wife, Julia,
whose enthusiastic support and encouragement
have aided me in the preparation of this book.

FOREWORD

The author, Harold Sheely Diehl, frankly disclaims the roles of disinterested observer and impartial reporter as he discusses tobacco and your health. But what must be said, and he is too modest to say it, is that three decades of concern about many health problems have led him to single out this one as paramount in our day.

For twenty-three years Harold Diehl was Dean of Medical Sciences and Professor of Public Health at the University of Minnesota. There, his broad interests and responsibilities made him aware of the whole gamut of human ills and of the effectiveness of our medical resources to deal with each of them. His experience led him to the conclusion that cancer and its allied diseases represent one of the major health problems that demand solution. So when he retired (in 1958) from the University of Minnesota, the American Cancer Society gained his services as Senior Vice-President for Research and Medical Affairs and Deputy Executive Vice-President.

During the past decade Dr. Diehl has focused his attention largely on smoking and health—cigarette smoking as related not only to cancer but to other serious diseases and disabilities as well. He has given leadership to the fight against this most formidable enemy. The battle involves changing a widespread and accepted social habit and also opposing the most powerful forces ever mobilized against efforts to reduce a public health hazard.

This book distills his wide experience into a powerful document to challenge the thoughtful reader, smoker and nonsmoker alike. It is no temperance tract, no emotional tirade, but a scientific book of fascinating fact that builds to an inescapable conclusion. The reader can see himself and his friends here. He is inspired to make personal decisions. He is guided by sound advice from doctors and psychologists. This book can save lives.

The objective assessment of the evidence presented here allows no halfway conclusions. Nor can the problems discussed be minimized. The least we can do is to be soundly informed on the subject.

Berwyn F. Mattison, M.D.
Executive Director, American Public Health Association

Why a book about tobacco and cigarette smoking? Reliable and authoritative books summarize and evaluate the evidence. Other books and many magazine articles consider efforts which are being made to reduce smoking and to assist smokers to give up the habit. Still others discuss the continuing efforts to persuade the public that smoking is a pleasurable, socially desirable, and harmless habit.

Surveys indicate that most people have heard of a relationship between cigarette smoking and cancer but that many of them consider the risk small and remote. Most people know little or nothing about the heart disease, the chronic bronchitis and emphysema, and the other illnesses that frequently result from smoking.

On a television news program in Phoenix, Arizona, I was asked: "What do you think of the reports that cigarette smoking causes lung cancer?" I replied that I was surprised that such a question would be asked in light of all the information on this subject which has been available to the public over the past fifteen years. The moderator's reply was: "This is a question that the public continues to ask." I found this hard to believe, but on reflection I realized that this question is not yet as fully answered in the minds of the public as I had thought.

The purpose of this book is to explore many of the questions concerning this problem that still trouble people—both smokers and non-smokers—and to give answers in the context of our complex society so that readers can take informed and meaningful action.

Dr. Charles A. Ross, Chief of the Thoracic Surgery Service of New York State's Roswell Park Memorial (Cancer) Institute, says: "Cigarette smoking is the most serious public health problem this country has ever faced." I agree with Dr. Ross, but I would add that it is also a most difficult, frustrating, and frequently discouraging problem. On the other hand, its importance is challenging and its story fascinating.

One major cause of public skepticism about the harmfulness of smoking has been the cleverness of advertising promoting the habit. Another cause has been the misleading propaganda of the cigarette industry. As an example of this: In January of 1968 more than a million persons in this country received copies of an article, reprinted from *True* magazine, entitled "To Smoke or Not to Smoke—That Is Still the Question." To each of these reprints was attached the statement: "As a leader in your profession and your community, you will be interested in reading this story— about one of today's controversial issues.—The Editors." A few months later a similar article appeared in a nationally distributed tabloid under the heading "Most Medical Authorities Agree— CIGARETTE LUNG CANCER LINK IS BUNK—70,000,000

Americans falsely alarmed." Both articles, it was later learned, were written by the same person, although under different names. Both articles were disguised propaganda for the tobacco industry's contention that "it has not been proved that cigarette smoking in any way impairs health." [1]

This book, *Tobacco and Your Health,* presents scientific and medically accepted information and judgment on this subject. As the author, I do not claim to be a disinterested, impartial observer or reporter. I have seen too much illness, disability, and premature death attributable to smoking to be that. On the other hand, I have attempted to maintain scientific objectivity. Any bias I may have is occasioned only by a desire to prevent some of the tragic results of cigarette smoking.

The decision *to smoke* or *not to smoke* must and should be made by each and every individual. It is my hope that this book will assist in the making of informed and wise decisions.

HAROLD S. DIEHL

[1] See pp. 217–230 for an analysis of these articles by The Wall Street Journal and the American Cancer Society.

ACKNOWLEDGMENTS

I wish to acknowledge and express appreciation for the encouragement, advice, and invaluable assistance in the preparation of this book that I have received from a number of scientists who have made distinguished contributions to our knowledge of the effects of tobacco on health, and from writers who have been leaders in interpreting to the public the results of this work. Prominent among these are James Monahan, Senior Editor, and Lois Mattox Miller, Roving Editor, of *Reader's Digest*; Dr. George E. Moore, Director of Research, Dr. Charles A. Ross, Chief of the Thoracic Surgery Service, and Dr. Ronald G. Vincent, Associate Chief of the Thoracic Surgery Service, of New York State's Roswell Park Memorial (Cancer) Institute, Buffalo, N.Y.; Dr. Daniel Horn, Director, and Emil Corwin, Information Officer, National Clearinghouse for Smoking and Health, U.S. Public Health Service; Dr. Ernest Wynder, Associate Member and Director, Division of

Experimental Carcinogenesis, Sloan-Kettering Institute for Cancer Research, New York City; Dr. James E. Perkins, Managing Director of the National Tuberculosis and Respiratory Disease Association; Dr. Oscar Auerbach, Senior Medical Investigator, Veterans Administration Hospital, East Orange, N.J.; and my colleagues on the staff of the American Cancer Society: Dr. E. Cuyler Hammond, Vice-President for Epidemiology and Statistics; Lawrence Garfinkel, Chief, Field and Special Projects, Epidemiology and Statistical Department; Edwin Silverberg, Project Statistician; Clifton R. Read, Senior Editor–Consultant, Secretary of the American Cancer Society Committee on Tobacco and Cancer; Theodore Adams, Director, Editorial Services; Walter G. James, Vice-President for Public Education; Dr. Sourya Henderson, Medical Librarian; and Miss Dorothy Nardecchia, my dedicated secretary.

HAROLD S. DIEHL

CONTENTS

RESPONSIBLE OPINIONS ABOUT TOBACCO & HEALTH

News items in the public press and on radio and television about the health hazards of cigarette smoking are commonly headlined as "the cigarette controversy" or "the smoking controversy." Public opinion polls indicate that a considerable proportion of the public accepts such statements as accurate. Yet there is no controversy or difference of opinion on this subject among medical and health organizations and agencies.

The Surgeon General of the U.S. Public Health Service says: "Cigarette smoking is the greatest preventable cause of illness, disability and premature death in this country."

The Commissioner of Health, State of New York, says: "No other single factor kills so many Americans as cigarette smoking. . . . Bullets, germs and viruses are killers; but for Americans, cigarettes are more deadly than any of them. No single known lethal agent is as deadly as the cigarette."

The Chief of the Thoracic Surgery Division of New York's Roswell Park Memorial (Cancer) Institute states: "Cigarette smoking is, without question, the greatest single public health problem this nation has ever faced."

The Director of Health of California has said:

> Cigarette smoking is one of the greatest threats to well being in modern times. Every appropriate preventive tool, every new, more effective method that can be devised, must be employed to stop this epidemic from spreading further among our young people, and roll it back from the adults. . . . It doesn't take long for this "social" habit to progress into full-fledged dependence. The boys and girls who become habituated are establishing an addiction that can kill or cripple them at a time when their rewards and contributions should be the greatest, with the loss not only theirs but society's as well.

The Association of State and Territorial Health Officers recommends

> that its members establish and carry out an effective program aimed at bringing under control the habit of cigarette smoking, thereby improving the health and well-being of the people of their states by reducing sickness, suffering, loss of earning power, and premature death.

At the World Conference on Smoking and Health, Sir George Godber, the Chief Medical Officer of the Ministry of Health of Great Britain, said:

> We can be certain that many more than 50,000 deaths a year in England and Wales are directly due to cigarette smoking and that of these deaths the number occurring before the age of 65 is sufficient to cause annually the loss at least of 150,000 years of working life. In addition to this there are the years of

progressive disability, so characteristic of chronic bronchitis that some people say that death from lung cancer is the lesser evil.

Similar statements have been made by the Ministers of Health of Canada, and of Norway, Sweden, Denmark, Russia, and other European countries.

The voluntary health organizations concerned with the diseases related to smoking have all taken clear-cut positions concerning the health hazards involved in cigarette smoking. The American Cancer Society says that "cigarette smoking is the major known cause of cancer deaths"; the American Heart Association that "cigarette smoking is a major factor in coronary heart disease" and that "the use of tobacco in all forms is a cause of peripheral vascular disease"—that is, spasms of and thrombus formation in the arteries of the legs and arms. The National Tuberculosis and Respiratory Disease Association has concluded that "the risk of disability from chronic bronchitis, emphysema, and certain other diseases is much greater among cigarette smokers than among nonsmokers." The American Medical Association has stated that "cigarette smoking is a serious health hazard." The American Public Health Association has made several statements on this subject, the latest being: "The health hazard of smoking is an accepted medical fact. . . . Immediate remedial action is essential to prevent thousands of unnecessary deaths."

The American College of Chest Physicians, the American College Health Association, the American Dental Association, the American Association for Thoracic Surgery, the American Academy of Pediatrics, the American Nurses Association, and many other national organizations and state and county medical societies have taken similar positions. The same is true of the Canadian Medical Association, the British Medical Association, the Royal College of Physicians of London, and many other responsible medical and health organizations in this country and abroad. In fact, no medical or health organization—not even a county medical society in "Marlboro Country"—has disagreed with these conclusions.

In September, 1967, the first World Conference on Smoking and Health was held in New York City. In his opening address the Chairman, Dr. Luther Terry, Vice-President–Medical Affairs, the University of Pennsylvania, Chairman of the National Interagency Council on Smoking and Health, and former Surgeon General of the U.S. Public Health Service, stated: "The period of uncertainty is over. There is no longer any doubt that cigarette smoking is a direct threat to the user's health. . . . Today we are on the threshold of a new era, a time of action, a time for public and private agencies, community groups and individual citizens to work together to bring this hydra-headed monster under control."

In spite of such total agreement among health and medical organizations, spokesmen for the tobacco interests keep saying: "There is no scientific proof that cigarette smoking causes any human disease or in any way impairs human health." In support of this theme cigarette advertisements imply that smoking is associated with robust health, vigor, charm, and romance.

How can there be such conflicting conclusions on a health issue of vital importance? And how can the public—both present smokers and individuals who have not started the habit—know what to accept as a basis for deciding whether to smoke or not to smoke?

So that each one may be able to make an intelligent decision on this question, we will present in subsequent chapters the evidence upon which one can base conclusions; the reasons *why* people smoke; the magnitude of the risk; dissenting opinions; and what is being done and what can be done about this health problem.

THE USE OF TOBACCO

In the late fifteenth century Columbus sailed westward from Spain hoping to bring back the riches of India. Instead he brought back tobacco—a plant that helped finance the Revolutionary War and for years proved to be America's most valuable export product. Columbus noted the use of tobacco by the natives of the islands he visited. These natives, whom he called Indians, smoked it in pipes for ceremonial purposes and as a symbol of goodwill.

The name "tobacco" was given this plant because of the Y-shaped pipe, called *tabaco*, in which it was sometimes smoked—one fork of the pipe being inserted into each nostril. Some pipes were made of baked clay, others of wood, others of soft, colorful rocks, many of which were artistically carved. In some areas Indians smoked tobacco rolled in the husks of corn.

The tobacco plant was later given the botanical name *nicotiana* in honor of Jean Nicot, the French Ambassador to Portugal, who is said to have sent seeds to the Queen of France, Catherine de' Medici.

TOBACCO—A MEDICINE

The Indians believed that tobacco had medicinal values. It was primarily for this reason that explorers took it back to Europe. About the middle of the seventeenth century a London doctor wrote a book entitled *Panacea; or the Universal Medicine, Being a Discovery of the Wonderful Vertues of Tobacco Taken in a Pipe, with Its Operation and Use both in Physick and Chyrurgery.* Among the "vertues" which he ascribed to tobacco were:

to cure deafness, a drop of the juice in each ear; to cure headache, a green tobacco leaf on the head; for redness of the face, apply the juice or the ointment of the tobacco leaf; for a toothache, tie a tobacco leaf over the aching region; for a cough, boil the leaves and shake the syrup on the stomach; for stomach pain and to take away the crudities of young and old, apply hot tobacco leaves over the region of the belly and re-heat whenever they get cool.

As if this were not an impressive enough list of "vertues," he goes on to recommend tobacco in the form of ointments, concoctions, powders, or leaves for burns, wounds, cancers, sciatica, diseases of the liver, of the spleen, of the womb, worms, colic, warts, corns, and mad dog bites.[1]

In spite of its presumed medicinal value, tobacco came into general use for quite different reasons. Sir Walter Raleigh is said to have promoted smoking in England. Of this Swinburne said: "James the First was a knave, a tyrant, a fool, a liar, a coward; but

[1] A. E. Hamilton, "This Smoking World," D. Appleton-Century Company, Inc., New York, 1927.

I love him, because he slit the throat of that blackguard Raleigh, who invented this filthy smoking."

THE USE OF TOBACCO
BECOMES WORLDWIDE

The smoking of tobacco in paper wrappers as small cigars or cigarettes originated in Spain in the seventeenth century. From Spain cigarettes spread eastward to Turkey and Russia and then westward to France and England, where they were introduced by soldiers who had served in Eastern Europe during the Crimean War.[2]

In London men who smoked cigarettes in public were at first ridiculed, but this was such a convenient way of smoking that it soon become popular on both sides of the Atlantic. The use of cigarettes received a great boost as they became better made and increasingly available with the development of improved methods of production.

Gradually the distribution and use of tobacco became worldwide, reaching even remote, undeveloped regions of Asia, Africa, and South America. A recent report by an anthropological research team states that in Columbia, South America, almost all the natives—men, women and children—even in primitive tribes in remote mountainous areas smoke tobacco. Such widespread distribution and use of a plant which until the past few centuries was limited to North America is an amazing phenomenon.

Tobacco exports now total about 600 million pounds annually of unmanufactured tobacco products, that is, tobacco leaf. Exported cigarettes make up about 5 percent of the total cigarettes manufactured, or about 116 billion cigarettes annually. U.S. export sales are

[2] Alfred Dunhill, ''The Gentle Art of Smoking,'' G. P. Putnam's Sons, New York, 1954.

promoted not only by tobacco company advertising but also by the U.S. Department of Agriculture, which does this to help dispose of the surplus stocks produced with the aid of government price supports.

Eighty-five percent of the tobacco produced in this country comes from the "tobacco belt," a region reaching north from Georgia to Kentucky and Virginia. In Virginia, North Carolina, South Carolina, and Kentucky tobacco is the single most valuable crop of the state; and in Tennessee, Georgia, Maryland, and Massachusetts it is the second largest in value. In 1966 tobacco contributed about $1.2 billion to farm income in the United States and about $6.6 billion to manufacturers' income.

Although the advertising and promotion of tobacco doubtless increases its use, no product would be so widely and universally accepted if it did not provide some satisfactions in the form of pleasure, stimulation, or gratification. Tobacco obviously does this for many smokers. The reasons will be considered in Chapter 11.

TABLE 2.1 Consumption of tobacco products per person aged 15 years and over in the United States for selected years, 1900–1967

Year	All tobacco, pounds	Cigarettes, number	Cigars, number	Pipe tobacco, pounds	Chewing tobacco, pounds	Snuff, pounds
1900	7.42	49	111	1.63	4.10	0.32
1910	8.59	138	113	2.58	3.99	0.50
1920	8.66	611	117	1.96	3.06	0.50
1930	8.88	1,365	72	1.87	1.90	0.46
1940	8.91	1,828	56	2.05	1.00	0.38
1950	11.59	3,322	50	0.94	0.78	0.36
1960	10.97	3,888	57	0.59	0.51	0.29
1965	10.78	3,982	65	0.54	0.49	0.23
1967	10.50	4,003	59	0.45	0.47	0.22

SOURCE: U.S. Department of Agriculture, Economic Research Service.

SNUFF

The most widespread and most ancient use of tobacco is for smoking. Columbus, however, noted that some Indians sniffed powdered tobacco through a tube. This form of tobacco was named snuff by the Dutch who promoted its use in Europe. Thought to have medicinal value, snuff was prescribed "to stop bleeding and to clear the head."

Snuff, although popular in Europe for centuries with all levels of society, was never widely used in this country. Currently it is consumed in the United States at the rate of about one-fifth of a pound per year per person over 15 years of age. This is about half the per capita consumption of 50 years ago.

CHEWING TOBACCO

Chewing tobacco, which consists of tobacco leaves mixed with molasses, was developed in this country and for years was used extensively. The amount of chewing tobacco sold in the United States at the beginning of this century averaged 4.1 pounds per person over 15 years of age. From this high its use has progressively declined, the spitoon has disappeared, and current use of chewing tobacco averages about one-half pound per person per year.

PIPE TOBACCO AND CIGARS

Pipe tobacco consumption remained relatively constant at two pounds per person from 1900 to 1940. Since 1940 its use has decreased greatly until it is now only about one-fifth what it was in 1940: 0.45 pound per person.

Crude cigars made of rolled tobacco leaves were smoked by natives of Cuba when this island was first visited by Columbus. Spanish and Portuguese sailors then started the making of cigars in their countries. Most cigar smokers consider cigar smoking the only real and civilized way to enjoy tobacco. Good cigars, however, are expensive, and their use decreased as first snuff, then pipes, and finally cigarettes became popular. In this country cigar smoking declined sharply between 1920 and 1930 when, as a by-product of World War I, cigarette smoking began to increase. In 1920 the average consumption per person 15 years of age and over was 117 cigars; by 1940 this figure had dropped 50 percent and has remained relatively constant at this level. In 1967 the average consumption of cigars and cigarellos per person 15 years and over in this country was 59.

CIGARETTES

Cigarette smoking prior to World War I was infrequent. A few brands were marketed but most smokers "rolled their own." Skill in rolling a good cigarette, particularly with one hand, was considered an art and a proud accomplishment. World War I with the free distribution of cigarettes to soldiers resulted in a tremendous increase in cigarette smoking. A second big increase followed the acceptance of cigarette smoking by women. Further increases occurred during World War II, the Korean War, and now the war in Vietnam.

Cigarettes are neatly packaged, convenient to carry, easily lit, and in most places socially acceptable. Cigarette smoke is relatively light and neutral, that is, neither acid nor alkaline. The great majority of cigarette smokers inhale to some degree and many inhale deeply. Generally, those who smoke most tend to inhale most deeply. On the other hand, few people can inhale the heavy and slightly alkaline smoke from cigars and pipes without coughing or becoming nauseated. Because of this, most cigar and pipe smokers inhale very little if at all.

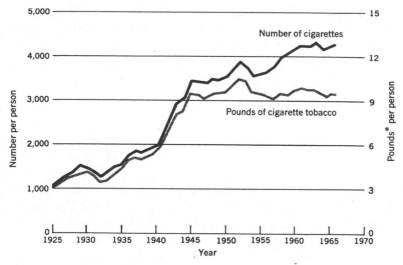

*Unstemmed processing weight of cigarette tobacco.

Figure 2.1. *Annual consumption of cigarettes per person 15 years or over, United States, 1925–1966. (Source: U.S. Department of Agriculture, "The Tobacco Situation.")*

In 1900 the average American 15 years of age and over smoked 49 cigarettes; in 1920, 611; in 1940, 1,828; in 1960, 3,888; in 1965, 3,982; and in 1967, 4,003. (See Table 2.1 and Figure 2.1.)

That the continuing increase in per capita consumption of cigarettes may be ending is suggested by a report in March, 1968, by Dr. Daniel Horn, director of the National Clearinghouse for Smoking and Health, which states that recent reports from the Internal Revenue Service show that for each of the three consecutive months of November, 1967, December, 1967, and January, 1968, there was an absolute reduction over the corresponding month a year earlier both in the manufacture of cigarettes and in the removal of cigarettes from warehouses for distribution to the consumer markets. This is the first time since shortly after the Surgeon General's Report of 1964 that such a continuing reduction has taken place.

The Department of Agriculture in March 1969 reported a decrease in domestic cigarette use for 1968 as compared to 1967 of 4.8 billion cigarettes. This decrease occurred despite a population increase of about 3 million. Per capita consumption by adults was about 2 per cent less in 1968 than in 1967. These figures do not include the armed services in which there was also a slight drop. (See page 207.)

FILTER–TIP CIGARETTES

Filter-tip cigarettes were first produced about 1950. In that year 0.5 percent of cigarettes sold were filter tip. In 1952, 1.3 percent of cigarettes produced were filter tip; in 1955, 19 percent; in 1960, 51 percent; in 1965, 64 percent; and in 1967, 70 percent.

The reason for the increasing sale of filter-tip cigarettes is the belief that filters remove at least some of the harmful ingredients in cigarette smoke. Laboratory studies show that this is true for some filter-tip cigarettes but not for all.

In some brands of cigarettes the amount of nicotine and tar is approximately four times as high as in others. This can be reduced by effective filters. However, the smoke of all cigarettes, even those with the best filters, contains substances which produce cancer in animals. Among filter-tip cigarettes some brands let through as much tar and nicotine (see page 201) as nonfilter cigarettes of the same brand. The President and Congress have said that the public has the right to know the amount of potentially harmful substances in the foods they eat and in the drugs they take. This should be true as well for the cigarettes they smoke. To provide this information the Federal Trade Commission has developed a laboratory to make official tests of the tar and nicotine content of cigarettes on the American market and is making the results of these tests available to the public. Bills have been introduced into the United States Congress to require that the tar and nicotine content of cigarettes be indicated on the packages and in cigarette advertising.

SMOKING BY WOMEN

Women rarely smoke pipes or cigars, and cigarette smoking by women did not become popular until the 1920s and 1930s. Until then very few women smoked, and smoking by women in public was almost unknown. The change was due in part to the increasing independence and freedom of women and their desire to do anything that men do. Probably an even greater factor was the tremendously skillful and intensive advertising campaign to make smoking by women socially acceptable and to associate smoking with characteristics that particularly appeal to women: romance, independence, glamour, and social success.

Cigarette advertisers got Metropolitan Opera stars to give testimonials for cigarettes, such as "Cigarettes are kind to your throat" and "I protect my voice with Lucky Strikes." Movie stars were shown smoking cigarettes and apparently enjoying it. Models in costumes of Lucky Strike green paraded up and down New York's Fifth Avenue smoking cigarettes. Sales promptly increased.

Then came the clever advertising slogan "Reach for a Lucky instead of a sweet." This was magic because most people, particularly women, have a fear of getting fat and know that candy is fattening. Sales of Lucky Strikes more than tripled within a year. No advertising campaign had ever been so successful.[3]

The large number of women smoking today conveys the impression that women are smoking as much as men, or even more. However, the American Cancer Society study of the smoking habits of some 440,000 men and 560,000 women shows that in the

[3] John Gunther, "Taken at the Flood—The Story of Albert Lasker," Harper and Brothers, New York, 1960, pp. 168–169.

age group 35 years and over, 47 percent of men smoke cigarettes compared with 27 percent of women, and that of those who smoke, 78 percent of men smoke a pack or more a day compared with 47 percent of women; also that 87 percent of the men smokers inhale moderately or deeply compared with 73 percent of women smokers; and that 73 percent of men started smoking before age 20 compared with 55 percent of women.[4]

In younger age groups the percentage of women who smoke more nearly approaches that of men. In future years, the effects of this increased smoking by women will most certainly be reflected in illness-, disability-, and death-rates.

[4] For a description of this study, see pp. 29–32.

SUSPICIONS & EARLY MEDICAL EVIDENCE

CHAPTER THREE

More than 300 years ago a Dr. Evard of London wrote:

> Young men must take great care how they suck this smoke for the custom and too much of it brings a grave out-of-order and makes them hot so that they lose their good temper and are beyond the bounds of health. Tobacco causes vomit and is an enemy of the stomach. Is it not a filthy thing and utterly to be detested that man, who is a most prudent creature, should be ensnared by the wanton enticement of this smoke of tobacco? . . . I think with Galen that it were better if any man have brains in his head to die a thousand times than to lead such a life.[1]

---

[1] A. E. Hamilton, "This Smoking World," D. Appleton-Century Company, Inc., New York, 1927.

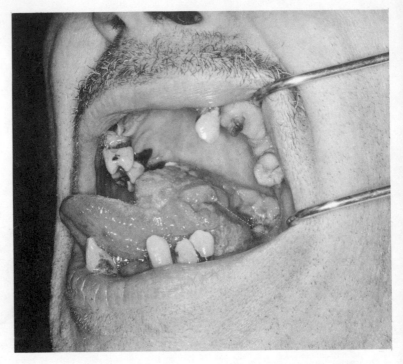

Figure 3.1. *Cancer of the tongue.* (*Courtesy Roswell Park Memorial Institute, Buffalo, N.Y.*)

SUSPICIONS OF
TOBACCO–CANCER
RELATIONSHIP

A century ago, Bouisson reported a remarkably thorough clinical study of 68 cases of cancer of the oral cavity in a hospital in France. Two-thirds of the cases were cancer of the lip, the others were cancer of the mouth, tongue, internal surface of the cheek, tonsil, and gum. Bouisson was able to ascertain the habits of 67 of these patients and found that 66 smoked tobacco and the other chewed tobacco. He noted, also, that cancer of the lip ordinarily occurred at the spot where the pipe or cigar was held.[2]

Also about a century ago, Oliver Wendell Holmes, author, poet and distinguished professor of the Harvard Medical School, wrote: "I think tobacco often does a great deal of harm to the health. I myself gave it up many years ago. I think self-narcotization is a rather ignoble substitute for undisturbed self." Similar opinions were expressed over the years by many physicians in this country and in Europe.

From time to time an apparent relationship of smoking to specific diseases, particularly lung cancer, was reported in medical journals. In 1927 an English physician, Dr. F. E. Tylecote, wrote that in almost every case of lung cancer he had seen or known about, the patient was a regular smoker, usually of cigarettes.

In 1936, Drs. Arkin and Wagner reported that of 135 men with lung cancer, 90 percent were "chronic smokers."[3]

At the International Cancer Congress in 1939, Dr. Alton Ochsner, a distinguished New Orleans surgeon, said: "It's our conviction that the increase in the incidence of pulmonary carcinoma is due largely to the increase in smoking, particularly cigarette smoking which is universally associated with inhalation."[4]

A few years later Dr. Ochsner commented upon the marked increase in patients with lung cancer and the fact that more than 95 percent of these patients were cigarette smokers. "During my medical student days," said Dr. Ochsner, "I saw only one lung

[2] M. Bouisson, "Du Cancer Buccal chez les Fumeurs," Montpelier Medical Journal, June and July, 1859.
[3] Aaron Arkin and David H. Wagner, "Primary Carcinoma of the Lung," Journal of the American Medical Association, vol. 106, p. 587, Feb. 22, 1936.
[4] Alton Ochsner, "Carcinoma of the Lung," Archives of Surgery, vol. 42, p. 209, February, 1941.

cancer case in four years. Today I operate on from two to five such cases every week. Now when I see a patient whose symptoms suggest lung cancer and who has been a heavy cigarette smoker, I make a tentative diagnosis of epidermoid lung cancer—or what has come to be known as Smoker's Cancer. Thus far I have been right in 98 percent of these diagnoses." [5]

EFFECTS OF SMOKING ON CIRCULATION

Early reports on the effects of tobacco upon the circulatory system were made by Drs. Irving S. Wright and Dean Moffat of New York and by Dr. Grace Roth of the Mayo Clinic, Rochester, Minnesota.[6] These studies reported that the smoking of a single cigarette causes a marked drop in the temperature of the fingers and toes. The subjects of these observations were confirmed smokers in average health. In a hundred cases the average drop was 5.3 F, the greatest drop 15.5°. Coincident with the drop in temperature a slowing or stopping of the blood flow in the capillaries frequently occurred. These changes occurred in experienced and heavy smokers as well as in light smokers and nonsmokers. The length of time a subject had smoked and the number of cigarettes habitually smoked daily had no effect on the temperature drop. The reason for the drop in temperature and for the blanching of skin is that smoking causes a constriction or spasm of the small arteries, called arterioles. This spasm narrows the lumen, i.e., the size of the opening within the vessels, thereby stopping or greatly reducing the flow of blood through the vessel. Some subjects showed marked toxic symptoms from smoking one cigarette. Others felt no or only slight symptoms from smoking. The infrequency of symptoms in experienced smokers is probably due to a

[5] Alton Ochsner, "Smoking and Cancer: A Doctor's Report," Julian Messner, Publishers, Inc., New York, 1954, p. 12.
[6] Irving S. Wright and Dean Moffat, "The Effects of Tobacco upon the Peripheral Vascular System," Journal of the American Medical Association, vol. 103, p. 319, Aug. 4, 1934; and Grace Roth, "Tobacco and the Cardiovascular System," Charles C. Thomas Publisher, Springfield, Ill., February, 1951.

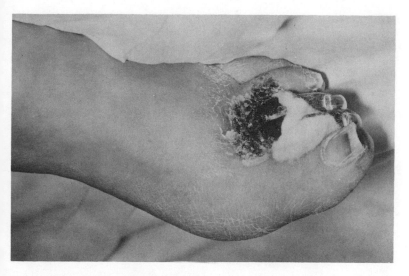

Figure 3.2. *Buerger's disease, with gangrene of the foot. (Courtesy Roswell Park Memorial Institute, Buffalo, N.Y.)*

conscious or unconscious control of the rate and depth of inhalation.

In some persons spasm of the small arteries is followed by the formation of a clot or *thrombus* within the vessel. This first reduces and then cuts off the flow of blood through the vessel. The condition is known as Buerger's disease. Gangrene may result and amputation of toes or fingers or even of legs or arms may be necessary. (See Figures 3.2 and 3.3.)

FIRST LONGEVITY TABLE OF SMOKERS

In 1938 Professor Raymond Pearl of Johns Hopkins University— the "father" of biostatistics in this country—published a life table on Smoking and the Length of Life. This was based upon the life histories of 6,813 men of whom 2,094 were nonusers of tobacco,

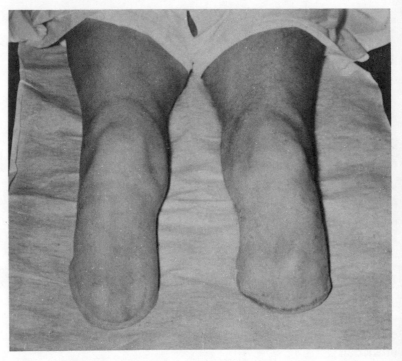

Figure 3.3. *Buerger's disease: bilateral amputation. (Courtesy Roswell Park Memorial Institute, Buffalo, N.Y.*

2,814 moderate smokers, and 1,905 heavy smokers. Dr. Pearl concluded that smoking is unquestionably associated with a definite reduction in the length of life and that the degree of reduction is proportional to amount of tobacco habitually used.[7] (Dr. Pearl's group of smokers included all smokers and did not differentiate between smokers of cigarettes, cigars, and pipes.)

As will be noted in Table 3.1, heavy smokers have the greatest reduction in the length of life but even moderate smoking is asso-

[7] Raymond Pearl, "The Search for Longevity," Scientific Monthly, vol. 46, pp. 462–483, May, 1938.

ciated with a significant reduction in life expectancy. This table shows also that during the important years between thirty and fifty the chances of a man's dying are 15 percent greater for a moderate smoker and 98 percent greater for a heavy smoker than for a nonsmoker. (Compare this early report by Dr. Pearl with the extensive study of this subject reported at the World Conference on Smoking and Health thirty years later; page 36.)

SMOKING AND LUNG CANCER

In 1930 a Dr. Muller of Cologne, Germany, compared the amount of smoking by 80 men with lung cancer with the smoking of 80 healthy men and found much more smoking among the cancer patients.

In 1944 Clarence Cook Little, Sc.D., the then managing director of the American Cancer Society, stated: "Although no definite evidence exists concerning the relation between the use of tobacco and the incidence of lung cancer, it would seem unwise to fill the

TABLE 3.1 Tobacco smoking and length of life*

Age	Nonusers	Moderate	Heavy	Age	Nonusers	Moderate	Heavy
30	100,000	100,000	100,000	65	57,018	52,082	38,328
35	95,883	95,804	90,943	70	45,919	41,431	30,393
40	91,546	90,883	81,191	75	33,767	30,455	22,338
45	86,730	85,129	71,665	80	21,737	19,945	14,498
50	81,160	78,436	62,699	85	11,597	10,987	7,865
55	74,538	70,712	54,277	90	4,573	4,686	3,392
60	66,564	61,911	46,226	95	1,320	1,366	938

* The number of survivors at 5-year intervals starting at the age of thirty of (1) 100,000 white males who were nonusers of tobacco, (2) 100,000 who were moderate smokers but did not chew tobacco or take snuff, and (3) 100,000 who were heavy smokers but did not chew or take snuff.

SOURCE: Raymond Pearl, "The Search for Longevity," Scientific Monthly, vol. 46, pp. 462–483, May, 1938.

lungs repeatedly with a suspension of fine particles of tobacco products of which smoke consists. It is difficult to see how such particles can be prevented from becoming lodged in the lungs and when so located how they can avoid producing a certain amount of irritation." [8]

In 1950 Drs. Ernest Wynder and Evarts Graham [9] of the Washington University School of Medicine in St. Louis investigated the smoking habits of 605 men with bronchogenic cancer of the lung other than adenocarcinoma and found that 96.5 percent of them had smoked at least half a pack of cigarettes a day for twenty years. Of these 605 lung cancer patients only 8 had been nonsmokers. Of the cancer group 51 percent were excessive or chain smokers as compared with 19 percent of male hospital patients without cancer. [10]

In 1952 Drs. Richard Doll and Bradford Hill of London published a careful study to evaluate reports of an association between smoking and cancer. They first located 709 hospitalized lung cancer patients and made a record of their smoking habits. They then located the same number of patients of the same age and sex who did not have lung cancer and recorded their smoking habits. Some of these "control" patients had cancer of other organs; some had other diseases. This study showed that there is a definite association between lung cancer and smoking, particularly cigarette smoking, and that a high proportion of the patients with lung cancer were heavy smokers. [11]

[8] C. C. Little, ''Cancer: A Study for Laymen,'' American Cancer Society, New York, 1944, p. 105.

[9] It was Dr. Graham, professor and head of the department of surgery, who performed in 1933 the first successful operation for the removal of a cancerous lung. His patient, a physician from Pittsburgh, lived and continued to practice medicine for many years thereafter.

[10] E. L. Wynder and Evarts A. Graham, ''Tobacco Smoking as a Possible Etiologic Factor in Bronchogenic Carcinoma: A Study of Six Hundred and Eighty Four Proved Cases,'' Journal of the American Medical Association, vol. 143, pp. 329–336, May 27, 1950.

[11] Richard Doll and A. B. Hill, ''A Study of the Etiology of Carcinoma of the Lung,'' British Medical Journal, vol. 2, p. 1271, Dec. 13, 1952.

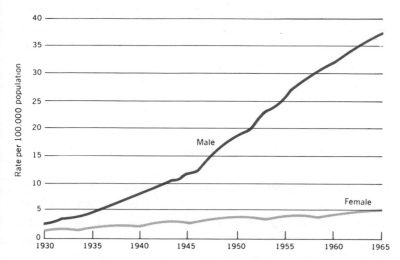

Figure 3.4. *Death rates for cancer of the lung by sex, United States, 1930–1965. (Source: American Cancer Society and U.S. Public Health Service.)*

Another somewhat different type of study was made of patients in hospitals owned and operated by the Seventh-Day Adventist religious group. These are excellent hospitals with competent staffs. They accept patients from the communities in which they are located whether or not they are members of the Seventh-Day Adventist church. The study compared the occurrence of lung cancer among patients who belong and those who do not belong to the Seventh-Day Adventist church. This comparison is clinically meaningful because members of this church are forbidden to use tobacco. The study revealed that patients who were not members of the church had about the amount of lung cancer one would expect in the general population. But among the Seventh-Day Adventists only two cases of lung cancer were found among the hundreds of patients cared for in these hospitals during the period of the study and both of these patients were recent converts to the church and previously had smoked a pack a day or more for many years.

Studies such as these look backward to investigate the smoking habits of patients with cancer or other diseases. They are therefore called "retrospective studies." If such studies show a consistent association between a disease and a possible cause, the conclusion is that the relationship is one of cause and effect, at least until proved otherwise.

Concerning cigarette smoking and lung cancer, twenty-nine retrospective studies involving more than 8,000 lung cancer patients in the United States, England, Germany, the Netherlands, Denmark, and other countries all reported similar conclusions. Practically all scientists, therefore, considered this conclusive evidence that cigarette smoking is a cause of lung cancer. However, to be doubly sure several investigators inaugurated the so-called prospective studies which will be considered in the next chapter.

PROSPECTIVE STUDIES—
GENERAL DEATH RATES

CHAPTER FOUR

Prospective studies record the smoking habits of large groups of individuals and obtain periodic reports, usually at yearly intervals, on subjects in the study who have died, together with the cause of death; these studies also record whether the individuals who are still living have been hospitalized and, if so, the cause. In cases of death, if an autopsy was performed, the cause of death given on the death certificate is verified or corrected. In regard to subjects who were hospitalized, information as to the cause of hospitalization is obtained from the patient, from the patient's physician, from the hospital, or from a member of the family. Since deaths and hospitalization increase with the passage of time, the longer the prospective study continues the greater its value.

After follow-up reports are received and entered on individual records, tabulations are made by groupings according to smoking

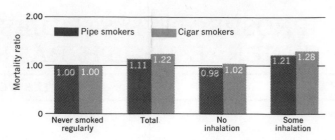

Figure 4.1. *Mortality ratios of male pipe and cigar smokers (age 45–54).* (*Source: American Cancer Society.*)

habits. Subgroups are then made by sex, age, and other factors concerning which information is desired, such as type of smoking, age at which smoking was started, inhalation, place of residence, occupation, etc.

The first of these prospective studies was by Drs. Doll and Hill of England, who sent a questionnaire about smoking habits to 60,000 British physicians aged 35 and over. From 40,000 of these physicians they obtained sufficient information to group them according to smoking habits. They received reports on these subjects for 4½ years and death certificates for those who had died. Analysis of these reports showed that "Mild smokers are seven times as likely to die of lung cancer as non-smokers; moderate smokers are 12 times as likely to die of lung cancer as non-smokers; immoderate smokers are 24 times as likely to die of lung cancer as non-smokers."[1]

At about the same time a much more extensive study was undertaken by Drs. E. Cuyler Hammond and Daniel Horn for the American Cancer Society. For this study 22,000 volunteers who had been trained as interviewers enrolled subjects in 394 counties in nine states between January 1 and May 31, 1952. The subjects,

[1] R. Doll and A. B. Hill, "Lung Cancer and Other Causes of Death in Relation to Smoking: A Second Report on the Mortality of British Doctors," British Medical Journal, vol. 2, p. 1071, 1956; and "Mortality in Relation to Smoking: Ten Years' Observation of British Doctors," British Medical Journal, vol. 1, pp. 1399 and 1460, 1964.

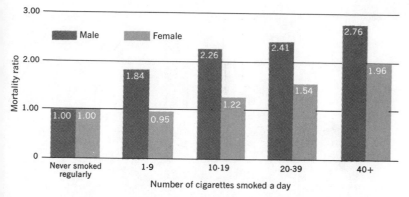

Figure 4.2. *Daily cigarette consumption and mortality ratios from all causes, by sex (age 45–54). (Source: American Cancer Society.)*

all of whom were men between the ages of 50 and 69, filled out a simple questionnaire relative to their smoking habits, both past and present. A total of 187,783 men were enrolled, filled out questionnaires, and were traced for the ensuing forty-four months. Death certificates were obtained on all who died, and additional medical information was obtained on those who were reported to have died of cancer. Altogether, 11,870 deaths were reported, of which 2,249 were attributed to cancer.

The most important findings of the study were that the total death rate, from all causes combined, is far higher among cigarette smokers than among nonsmokers or pipe and cigar smokers and that the death rate increases in direct relation to the number of cigarettes smoked.[2]

Another prospective study was carried out by Dr. Harold F. Dorn of the U.S. Public Health Service. After determining the smoking habits of 200,000 veterans holding government life insurance poli-

[2] E. C. Hammond and Daniel Horn, "Smoking and Death Rates: Report on 44 Months of Follow-up on 187,783 Men," Journal of the American Medical Association, vol. 166, pp. 1159 and 1294, 1958.

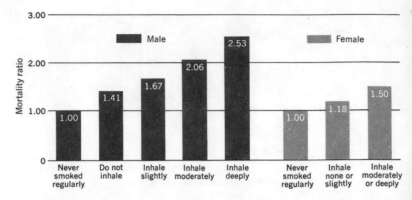

Figure 4.3. *Inhalation and mortality ratios, all causes, of cigarette smokers, by sex (age 45–54). (Source: American Cancer Society.)*

cies, he then noted the causes of deaths in this group over a period of 2½ years. His conclusion was that in this group cigarette smokers were 10 times as likely to die of lung cancer as nonsmokers and that men who smoke more than a pack a day were 16 times as likely to die from lung cancer as nonsmokers.[3] Similar studies of Canadian veterans gave comparable results.[4]

The two most recent and largest prospective studies of the relationship between cigarette smoking and lung cancer were conducted by H. A. Kahn of the U.S. Public Health Service and Dr. E. Cuyler Hammond for the American Cancer Society.

Mr. Kahn continued Dr. Dorn's study for 8½ years. He concluded that the increased mortality risk associated with cigarette smoking was higher in the more recent time period than in the initial years of study.[5]

[3] H. F. Dorn, "Tobacco Consumption and Mortality from Cancer and Other Diseases," Public Health Reports, vol. 74, p. 581, 1959.
[4] E. W. R. Best, "A Canadian Study of Smoking and Health," Department of Health and Welfare, Ottawa, Canada, 1966.
[5] H. A. Kahn, "The Dorn Study of Smoking and Mortality Among U.S. Veterans: Report on 8½ Years of Observation," National Cancer Institute Monograph, no. 19, January, 1966, pp. 1–125.

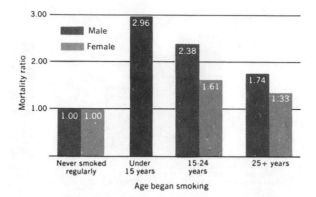

Figure 4.4. *Age of beginning to smoke and mortality ratios, by sex.* Note: No "Under 15 years" bar is included for females because the number of deaths in that age group does not offer a sufficient basis for the computation of a reliable mortality ratio. (*Source: American Cancer Society.*)

Dr. Hammond's most recent study was started in 1959 and involved more than a million subjects—440,558 men and 562,671 women—in 1,121 counties in twenty-five states. The follow-up covered four years. Conclusions concerning the overall death rate were as follows:

Death rates of both men and women were higher among subjects with a history of cigarette smoking than among those who never smoked regularly. Death rates of current cigarette smokers increased with the number of cigarettes smoked per day and the degree of inhalation.

Death rates were higher among current cigarette smokers who started the habit at a young age than among those who started later in life. Among both men and women, the difference between the death rates of cigarette smokers and nonsmokers increased with age.

Among men, the death rates for ex-cigarette smokers were lower than for men smoking cigarettes when they enrolled in the study.

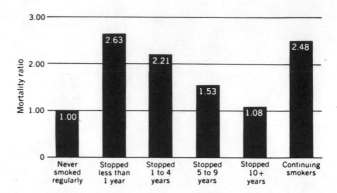

Figure 4.5. *Mortality ratios of male ex-cigarette smokers (age 45–54).* *(Source: American Cancer Society.)*

The death rates of ex-cigarette smokers decreased with the length of time since they last smoked cigarettes. (Figure 4.5.)

Total death rates and death rates from most of the common diseases occurring in both sexes were higher for men than for women, higher for men who never smoked regularly than for women who never smoked regularly, and far higher for men who were regular cigarette smokers than for women who smoked regularly.

Among both men and women, death rates from the following diseases were much higher in cigarette smokers than in non-smokers: emphysema; cancer of the lung; cancer of the buccal cavity (i.e., tissues inside of the mouth); cancer of the pharynx, larynx, and esophagus; aortic aneurysm; and cancer of the pancreas. (Figure 4.6.)

Death rates from coronary heart disease and from strokes also were significantly higher—about twice as high—for both men and women who smoked than for nonsmokers.

The difference between the death rates of subjects with a history of cigarette smoking and subjects who never smoked regularly was

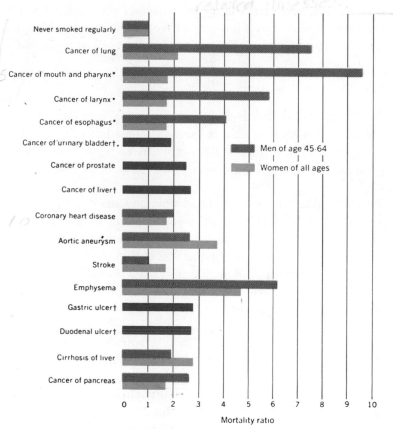

Figure 4.6. *Major causes of death among cigarette smokers as compared with nonsmokers, by sex. (Source: American Cancer Society.)*

*Because of small number of these cancers in groups of women studied, these cancers were combined in computing mortality ratios.

†Because of small numbers of deaths from these causes among women studied, mortality rates were not computed.

much greater among men than among women. Female cigarette smokers (as a group) have been far less exposed to cigarette smoke than male cigarette smokers of the same ages, as judged by the number of cigarettes smoked per day, the degree of inhalation, and the number of years they have smoked. Many female cigarette

smokers smoke only a few cigarettes a day, do not inhale, and have
been smoking for only a few years; their death rates are about the
same as the death rates of women who never smoked regularly.[6]

Matched pair analysis

Critics of studies which show an association between cigarette
smoking and disease insist that there may be a factor, a genetic or
individual characteristic, which occurs in cigarette smokers and
predisposes them to lung cancer and certain other diseases.

To investigate this assertion Dr. Hammond made a unique and
significant study of 442,049 men whose smoking habits and condition of health were followed for an average of 34.3 months.[7] By
use of a computer Dr. Hammond was able to find in this group
36,975 "matched pairs" of men in which one member of each pair
smoked a pack or more of cigarettes daily while the other member
had never smoked regularly.

The characteristics matched in these groups were: race (white,
Negro, Mexican, Indian, or Oriental); height; nativity (native-
born or foreign-born); residence (rural or urban); urban occupational exposure to dusts, fumes, vapors, chemicals, radioactivity,
etc.; religion (Protestant, Catholic, Jewish, or none); education;
marital state; consumption of alcoholic beverages; amount of sleep
per night; usual amount of exercise; nervous tension; use of
tranquilizers; current state of health; history of cancer other than
skin cancer; and history of heart disease, stroke, or high blood
pressure.   -

Thus each pair had the same characteristics except that one man
of each pair smoked and the other did not. The analysis of these

[6] E. C. Hammond, "Smoking in Relation to the Death Rates of One Million Men
and Women," National Cancer Institute, Monograph 19, Jan., 1966, pp. 127–204.
[7] E. Cuyler Hammond, "Smoking in Relation to Mortality and Morbidity," Journal
of the National Cancer Institute, U.S. Public Health Service, Washington, vol. 32,
no. 5, pp. 1161–1187, May, 1964.

36,975 nonsmokers and 36,975 smokers over this period of about three years showed that:

1   A total of 1,385 (3.7 percent) of the cigarette smokers died compared with 662 (1.8 percent) of the nonsmokers.

2   110 smokers died of lung cancer compared with only 12 nonsmokers.

3   12 smokers died of cancer of the buccal cavity, pharynx, larynx, and esophagus compared with 1 nonsmoker.

4   23 smokers died of cancer of the pancreas and liver compared with 7 nonsmokers.

5   15 smokers died of emphysema compared with only 1 nonsmoker.

6   30 smokers died of aortic aneurysm compared with 8 nonsmokers.

7   654 smokers died of coronary heart disease compared with 304 nonsmokers.

The conclusions to be drawn from such results are obvious to anyone. For a complete tabulation of the analyses of this study, see Appendix B, pages 215, 216.

NUMBER OF DEATHS
ATTRIBUTABLE TO SMOKING

In 1965 Dr. Luther Terry, the Surgeon General of the U.S. Public Health Service, stated: [8]

> Studies of mortality ratios of smokers and non-smokers indicate that 240,000 men will this year die prematurely from diseases associated with cigarette smoking. About 138,000 of these excess or premature deaths will be from diseases clearly and definitely associated with smoking, such as cancer of the

[8] Luther Terry, ''Emerging Anti-Smoking Activities of the Federal Government,'' Address at Annual Meeting of the National Tuberculosis Association, Chicago, Ill., May 31, 1965.

lung, larynx, oral cavity, esophagus and bladder, as well as bronchitis, emphysema and coronary heart disease. Another 102,000 excess or premature deaths will result from diseases where the relationship to cigarette smoking, while not so obvious, is nevertheless clearly indicated.

This total of 240,000 premature deaths applies to men only, because in most cases the data for women are inadequate to make precise estimates. Where data are available for women, mortality ratios for comparable levels of smoking appear to be similar to those for men, but somewhat lower. A reasonable estimate of excess deaths among women, added to the total of 240,000 for men, would bring the over-all total to 300,000. I consider this total to be a reasonable estimate.

In 1967 the current Surgeon General, Dr. William H. Stewart, stated that the number of deaths attributable to smoking was in excess of 300,000.

A similar estimate was made at the World Conference on Smoking and Health by Dr. R. T. Ravenholt, Professor of Preventive Medicine at the University of Washington and Director of Population Service of the U.S. Agency for International Development. Dr. Ravenholt presented a Balance Sheet of Hazards to Life in 1966. (Table 4.1)

Translated into daily averages these figures mean that approximately 800 deaths a day in this country are attributable to cigarette smoking. Of these about 175 a day are due to cancer; 375 a day to diseases of the heart and circulatory system; and 250 a day to chronic bronchitis, emphysema, peptic ulcers, and other diseases.

CIGAR AND PIPE SMOKING

Studies also show some relationship of cigar and pipe smoking to coronary heart disease, peripheral vascular disease, and cancers of the mouth, the pharynx, and the larynx. However, these diseases are less closely related to cigar and pipe smoking than to cigarette smoking.

TABLE 4.1 An American balance of hazards to life, 1966

Excess Deaths from Tobacco *

Lung cancer	41,012
Other cancers (of larynx, bladder, etc.)	28,045
Coronary disease	145,956
Other vascular diseases (strokes, etc.)	42,821
All other causes (emphysema, bronchitis, etc.)	43,726
Excess deaths from tobacco	301,560

Deaths from Selected Causes

All infections	128,180
Tuberculosis	(7,590)
Pneumonia and influenza	(64,230)
All accidents	112,300
Motor vehicle	(53,280)
Diabetes	35,380
Suicide	20,160
Homicide	11,210
Balancing total	307,310

SOURCE: R. T. Ravenholt: Presented at World Conference on Smoking and Health, September, 1967.

The overall death rate is also much less affected by cigar and pipe smoking than by cigarette smoking. For men who smoke only cigars the death rate is 22 percent higher than that of nonsmokers between the ages of 45 and 64, and 5 percent higher for men over 65. For pipe smokers, the mortality rate is 11 percent higher than for nonsmokers between 45 and 64 and 2 percent higher for those over 65.

SMOKING AND THE LENGTH OF LIFE

Another measure of the hazard of smoking is its relationship to the length of life. Dr. Raymond Pearl's 1938 report showed this relationship at that time (see page 19). A vastly more extensive study was presented to the World Conference on Smoking and Health in 1967 by Dr. Hammond of the American Cancer Society. For this study, tables were developed which show the life expectancy of cigarette smokers and nonsmokers at various ages. Table 4.2 shows the remaining years of life at given ages in relation to cigarette smoking. The study also shows that the life expectancy of a man 25 years of age is reduced by 4.6 years if he smokes less than a half a pack of cigarettes a day; by 5.5 years if he smokes ½ to 1 pack a day; by 6.2 years if he smokes 1 to 2 packs a day; and by 8.3 years if he smokes 2 or more packs a day. Comparable data covering smoking habits and death rates of women were not adequate to prepare similar life expectancy tables.

TABLE 4.2 **Life expectancy and cigarette smoking (estimate for United States males)**

| | Remaining life expectancy in years | | | | |
| | Never smoked regularly | Cigarette smokers by daily amount | | | |
Age		1–9	10–19	20–39	40+
25	48.6	44.0	43.1	42.4	40.3
30	43.9	39.3	38.4	37.8	35.8
35	39.2	34.7	33.8	33.2	31.3
40	34.5	30.2	29.3	28.7	26.9
45	30.0	25.9	25.0	24.4	23.0
50	25.6	21.8	21.0	20.5	19.3
55	21.4	17.9	17.4	17.0	16.0
60	17.6	14.5	14.1	13.7	13.2
65	14.1	11.3	11.2	11.0	10.7

SOURCE: E. C. Hammond: "World Costs of Cigarette Smoking in Disease, Disability, and Death," World Conference on Smoking and Health, New York, September 11, 1967.

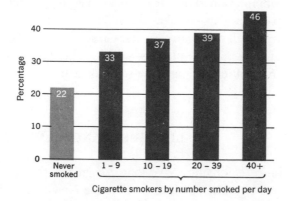

Cigarette smokers by number smoked per day

Figure 4.7. *Percentage of males aged 25 expected to die before 65, in relation to cigarette smoking. (Source: E. C. Hammond, "Life Expectancy of American Men in Relation to their Smoking Habits." Based on data from American Cancer Society Cancer Prevention Study presented at World Conference on Smoking and Health, N.Y., Sept. 11, 1967.)*

Incidentally, but of great significance, the *decrease* in life expectancy of the two-pack-a-day smoker is almost equal to the *increase* in life expectancy over the past fifty years. Thus, heavy cigarette smokers sacrifice for smoking all the health gains made over the past half century not only by the advances in medical science but also by improvements in nutrition and in the social and economic conditions of life.

Another way of presenting the effect of smoking upon longevity is graphically shown in Figure 4.7. Thus the chances of a man aged 25 dying before 65—the peak years of his family and professional or business responsibilities—are 50 percent greater for one who smokes less than half a pack of cigarettes a day than for a non-smoker; 70 percent greater for one who smokes one-half to one pack a day; 77 percent greater for one who smokes one to two packs a day; and 109 percent greater (more than twice as great) for one who smokes two or more packs a day.

Another computation shows that the average heavy smoker—two or more packs a day—smokes during his lifetime about three-quarters of a million cigarettes. As a result of this he loses 8.3 years—about 4.4 million minutes—of life. This amounts to a loss of almost 6 minutes per cigarette smoked: a minute of life for a minute of smoking.

LIFE INSURANCE AND SMOKING

Life insurance companies have long recognized the risk of early death among cigarette smokers. In fact, the New England Mutual Life Insurance Company in 1911 made an analysis of the relation of the use of tobacco to mortality. The study covered sixty years

TABLE 4.3 Percentage of men aged 25 surviving at 5-year intervals in relation to age they began cigarette smoking (based upon rates adjusted to the 1959–1961 U.S. life table for all males)

Age	All men	Never smoked regularly	Age began cigarette smoking			
			25–34	20–24	15–19	<15
25	100.0	100.0	100.0	100.0	100.0	100.0
30	99.1	99.4	99.4	99.3	99.1	98.8
35	98.2	98.7	98.6	98.3	98.1	97.3
40	96.8	97.8	97.6	97.0	96.6	95.2
45	94.6	96.4	95.8	95.0	93.7	91.5
50	91.1	94.4	92.5	91.1	88.9	86.4
55	85.6	90.9	87.4	84.9	82.0	78.4
60	78.1	85.5	79.2	76.8	72.7	67.7
65	67.8	77.7	67.2	65.0	60.2	55.5
70	55.2	66.7	52.5	50.8	44.7	39.7
75	41.2	52.3	38.7	35.1	30.0	24.6
80	26.7	35.6	24.6	20.4	16.8	14.0
85	13.6	19.2	10.5	9.1	6.3	5.8
90	4.9	7.0	3.8	2.8	1.4	1.5
95	1.0	1.5	0.8	0.6	0.3	0.3

SOURCE: . See footnote, Table 4.2, p. 36.

and a total of 130,000 policy holders. The conclusions were that men who "rarely" used tobacco had a 25 percent greater mortality than men who did not use tobacco at all; that "temperate" users of tobacco showed a 45 percent and "moderate" users a 61 percent increased mortality.[9]

Since then insurance companies have taken this risk into consideration in connection with applications for large policies, usually not directly but rather by giving special attention to pulse rate, blood pressure, cough, diminished lung capacity, etc.

In recent years several insurance companies have been offering life insurance at reduced rates to those who do not smoke cigarettes. Cigar and pipe smokers are usually considered as nonsmokers for insurance purposes. The reason that all companies do not do this is that it is easier to continue to charge excessive rates to non-smokers to offset the high mortality risk of smokers than it is to charge smokers the higher rates that their greater risk of early death would justify.

[9] Personal communication from Dr. Richard B. Singer, medical director.

SUBSTANCES IN TOBACCO SMOKE & THEIR IMMEDIATE EFFECTS

CHAPTER FIVE

Tobacco smoke is a mixture of gases, vapors, and chemical compounds. The relative amount of each depends upon the type of tobacco, the way it is smoked, and the temperature at which it is burned. The higher the temperature, the greater amount of these substances produced. While air is being drawn through a cigarette, the temperature of the burning zone reaches approximately 880°C.

The potentially harmful gases in cigarette smoke include carbon monoxide in a concentration 400 times that considered a safe level in industrial exposure and hydrogen cyanide in a concentration 160 times the amount considered safe in industry. Hydrogen cyanide is a powerful poison.

Carbon monoxide, the deadly gas from automobile exhausts, combines with hemoglobin in red blood cells, thereby reducing the

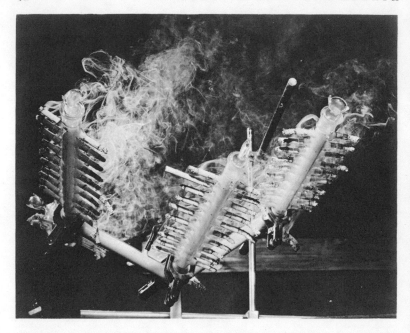

Figure 5.1. A "smoking robot," simulating the smoking manner of humans, puffs away on unevenly burning cigarettes. This automatic device, which lights its cigarettes simultaneously, uniformly "inhales" a predetermined amount of smoke, thus affording a controllable and equitable means of trapping tars. (Courtesy American Cancer Society.)

oxygen-carrying capacity of the blood. In the blood of an average smoker 2 to 6 percent of the hemoglobin is inactivated by carbon monoxide and in a heavy smoker up to 8 percent. Since carbon monoxide has a much greater affinity for hemoglobin than does oxygen, it literally drives oxygen from the blood. This reduction of available oxygen decreases one's ability to perform strenuous activity and makes smokers "short of breath" upon exertion. Carbon monoxide also decreases one's tolerance to high altitudes and has an effect upon the sensitivity of the eye, particularly at night. If carbon monoxide levels in the blood reach 30 percent, serious illness results. At levels above 60 percent death occurs (page 53).

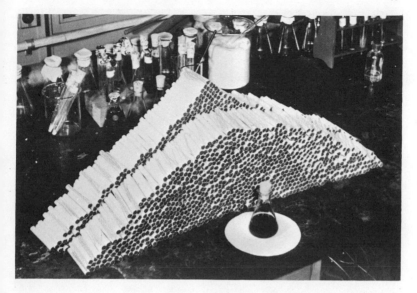

Figure 5.2. *These 2,000 cigarettes will produce the amount of tobacco tar shown in the flask in the foreground. (Courtesy American Cancer Society.)*

Several hundred different chemicals make up the so-called particulate matter or tiny particles in tobacco smoke. There are millions or even billions of these per cubic centimeter of smoke. This particulate matter when condensed forms the brown, sticky mass called *tobacco tar* or cigarette tar. It can be seen around the exhausts of the ventilating systems of airplanes or by blowing smoke through a handkerchief. These tars contain nicotine and more than a dozen chemicals that produce cancer when applied to the skin or bronchi of mice or other laboratory animals. Such chemicals are called *carcinogenic*, meaning cancer-producing.

The smoking machine shown in Figure 5.1 is in use at the Roswell Park Memorial (Cancer) Institute at Buffalo, New York. It smokes 20,000 cigarettes a day, 600 at a time. It loads and lights itself, inhales five times, knocks off the ash, inhales five more times, spits out the cigarette, then loads itself again. This con-

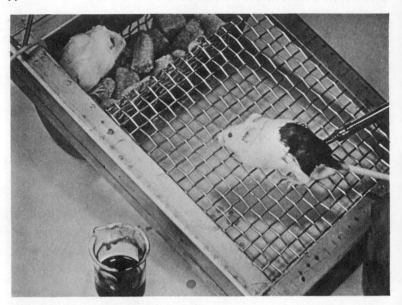

Figure 5.3. *Painting the skin of a mouse with tar from cigarette smoke.*
(Courtesy Roswell Park Memorial Institute, Buffalo, N.Y.)

tinues all day, and at the end of the day this machine will have collected three-fourths of a pound of tar from the smoke of the cigarettes.

If a dilute solution of this tar, from just a few packages of cigarettes, is painted repeatedly on the skin of small animals, 60 percent of these animals will develop cancers of the skin within a year.

Chemical analysis of tobacco tar shows that it contains more than 200 compounds, many of them toxic. Among these are at least 10 hydrocarbons that produce cancer in animals. If a 1 to 1,000 dilution of just one of these chemicals, known as benzpyrene, is placed in paraffin pellets and if one of these pellets is implanted in the cheek pouch of a hamster for a period of twenty-five weeks, 90 percent of these animals will develop cancer of the mouth.

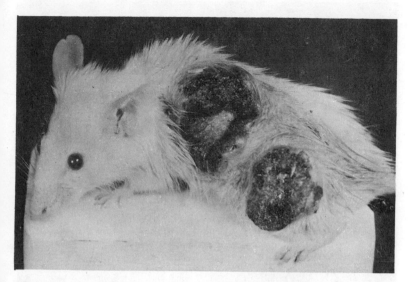

Figure 5.4. *Cancers of the skin of a mouse, caused by painting with tobacco tars. (Courtesy Roswell Park Memorial Institute, Buffalo, N.Y.)*

Nicotine is a colorless, oily compound which in concentrated form is one of the most powerful poisons known. It has no medical use but is marketed as an insecticide under the name of Black Leaf 40. The injection of one drop, 70 milligrams, will cause the death of a man of average weight within a few minutes. The same amount placed on the gum of a dog will kill the dog. The nicotine content of cigarettes sold in this country ranges from about 0.5 milligrams per cigarette in some brands to 2 milligrams in others.

Certain chemicals in tobacco tar, called *co-carcinogens*, do not produce cancers themselves but act with other chemicals to stimulate the growth of certain cancers. Others, called *phenols*, first stop and then destroy the protective action of the cilia—the small hair-like projections—that line the respiratory tract. Still others are irritants which cause the so-called cigarette cough and probably are responsible for the gradual destruction of lung tissue that results in emphysema. Every smoker absorbs some of the nicotine and the

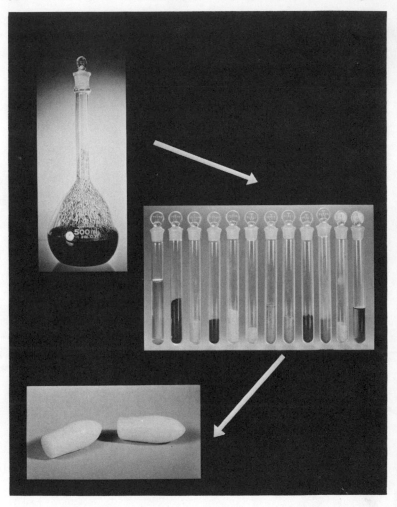

Figure 5.5. Top: *flask of tobacco tar.* Middle: *chemical fractions of tobacco tar.* Bottom: *paraffin pellets containing benzpyrene from tobacco tar.* (*Courtesy Roswell Park Memorial Institute, Buffalo, N.Y.*)

tars in cigarette smoke. Those who inhale retain most of these substances in the body. However, in cigar and cigarette smoking the tobacco acts to filter out and to retain some of the tar and nicotine in the smoke. For this reason the amount taken into the

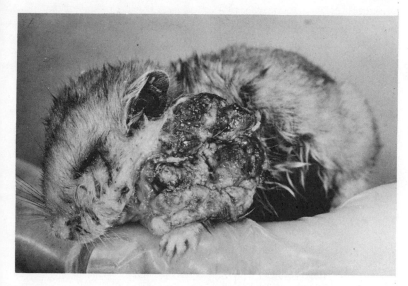

Figure 5.6. *Hamster with cancer from implantation of benzpyrene pellet.* (Courtesy Roswell Park Memorial Institute, Buffalo, N.Y.)

body in smoking the last third of a cigarette is several times the amount from the first third.

IMMEDIATE EFFECTS OF SMOKING

The beginning smoker often has symptoms of mild nicotine poisoning. Even habitual smokers sometimes show the same effects. These symptoms include dizziness, faintness, rapid pulse, cold, clammy skin, and sometimes nausea, vomiting, and diarrhea.

In most people, smoking reduces the appetite and dulls the sense of taste and smell. The unattractive brown stains left on the teeth and fingers of cigarette smokers are caused by tobacco tars. Both nicotine and tobacco tars are irritating. The tars are responsible for the loss of smell, for unpleasant mouth conditions, and for the malodorous breath of smokers.

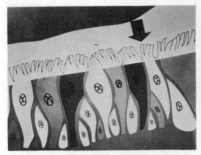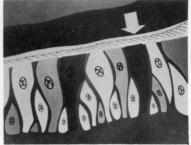

Figure 5.7. *Bronchial cilia, an important part of the body's filtering mechanism, are immobilized by continued cigarette smoking. Left: the arrow points to the normal appearance of cilia—tiny, hair-like structures which serve to keep foreign particles from entering the lungs. Right: with cilia weakened, the bronchus has difficulty in getting rid of mucus, which builds up. This produces the well-known "smoker's cough," as the bronchus is forced to exert unusual effort in order to expel the mucus. (Courtesy American Cancer Society.)*

On digestion

A cigar, a cigarette, or a pipe after meals may give the habitual smoker a certain comfortable and satisfied feeling. On the other hand, the use of tobacco may give rise to various chronic digestive disturbances. Several studies have shown that ulcers of the stomach are five times as frequent and ulcers of the duodenum twice as frequent in cigarette smokers as in nonsmokers and that cancer of the stomach is 40 percent more likely to develop in smokers than in nonsmokers.

On the nervous system

The most notable effect of nicotine is a transient stimulation followed by depression of both the sympathetic and the central nervous systems. Nicotine also causes a discharge of epinephrine from the adrenal glands. This in turn stimulates the nervous system and other endocrine glands and causes the release of glycogen (sugar) from the liver. The result is a feeling of stimulation or "kick" and relief of fatigue. This, however, is transient and is followed by depression and further fatigue. Nicotine is believed to be the addictive ingredient of tobacco.

On the respiratory system

Tobacco smoke contains substances which irritate the mucus membrane of the respiratory tract; and it is well known that excessive smoking causes cough, hoarseness, bronchitis, and other related conditions. "Smoker's throat," "smoker's larynx," "smoker's cough," and "smoker's bronchitis" have for years been common terms. These symptoms usually disappear when one stops smoking.

The bronchial tubes of the lungs have a remarkable protective mechanism. The cells lining these tubes and tubules secrete mucus, a sticky fluid which collects particles of soot, dust, and other substances in inhaled air. This mucus is carried up through the bronchial tubes and the trachea by the action of the cilia and is either swallowed or expectorated. These cilia are little hairlike structures which protrude from the inner surface of the respiratory passages and maintain a continuous whiplike motion of about 900 beats a minute. Their movement causes mucus to flow up and out of the lungs. Particles of inhaled dust and other substances trapped in the mucus are thus removed, keeping the lungs clean and protecting the bronchial tubes from damage. If the pollution of the inhaled air is more than this system can remove, or if the cilia are destroyed or fail to work, this protection is lost. Cigarette smoke first slows, then stops ciliary action and eventually destroys the cilia, thereby exposing delicate membranes to injury by substances inhaled in cigarette smoke or in the air we breathe.

An analysis of respiratory diseases among 179 boys 14 to 19 years of age in a New Jersey preparatory school showed that severe respiratory illnesses were nine times as frequent among regular smokers as among nonsmokers. Among occasional smokers, these illnesses were 2.6 times as common as among nonsmokers.

These findings are consistent with the statement by nose and throat specialists that they can easily identify a smoker by the irritated, inflamed appearance of the mucous membranes of the nose and pharynx.

On circulation

The heart rate increases after smoking. In one group of young people studied, the average increase after a single cigarette was twenty-one beats per minute. Occasionally, the heartbeat becomes irregular and there is pain in the chest. Blood pressure usually rises and may remain elevated for some time.

Smoking causes the small arteries to contract, or become smaller. This cuts down the flow of blood through these vessels and results in a lowering of the temperature of the skin. This occurs in habitual smokers as well as in beginners. In a study of 100 persons, the smoking of a single cigarette caused an average drop of 5.3° F in the temperature of the fingers and toes.

The immediate effects of smoking were further investigated in 1967 at the San Fernando State College in California with 400 male students as subjects. It was noted that during smoking the heart rate and the systolic blood pressure increase and abnormal changes occur in the electrocardiogram. There was also an indication that blood clotted faster after one had smoked a cigarette and that smokers were less efficient than nonsmokers in their work tasks.

On fatigue

Some people think that tobacco relieves fatigue. This may be because nicotine causes a temporary increase of sugar in the blood, and more sugar means more fuel for the muscles. After a brief time, however, the fuel is used up and the feeling of fatigue is greater than before. It is also said that smoking relaxes nervous tension. This is doubtless true for habituated smokers whose craving for a smoke is relieved by a cigarette. There is no evidence that cigarette smoking has any other tranquilizing effects.

On the endocrine system

Various studies have shown that cigarette smoking or the injection of nicotine stimulates the adrenal gland to produce increased amounts of hormones which affect the action of other organs and other glands of internal secretion. A recent study was reported from the Philadelphia General Hospital in which five men and four women ranging in age from 22 to 30 years, all chronic smokers, participated. After they had smoked cigarettes in the normal manner for 30 minutes, blood samples were taken and analyzed. The result showed an increase of from 27 to 77 percent in the amount of adrenal hormones in the blood. The average rise was 47 percent. By contrast a group of control subjects who had not smoked showed a decline in these hormones, which normally vary according to the time of day. The one subject who smoked cigars and a pipe instead of cigarettes showed no rise in hormone level.

In other experiments, dogs and rats were given nicotine internally. This resulted in hormone increases comparable to those found in the human subjects.

The physicians who made this study did not suggest what effects, if any, the smoking hormone link might have on health. However, the clear implication was that any unnatural change in the normal amount of essential hormones could be harmful.[1]

[1] Alfred Kershbaum, M.D., et al., "Effect of Smoking and Nicotine on Adrenocortical Secretion," Journal of the American Medical Association, vol. 203, pp. 275–278, Jan. 22, 1968.

On endurance

The effect of cigarette smoking on endurance performance was measured in 419 airmen before and after six weeks of basic training at the U.S. Air Force Aerospace Medical Laboratory, Lackland Air Force Base, Texas. Field testing showed that endurance was inversely related to the number of cigarettes smoked daily and the duration of smoking. The beneficial effects of training were significantly reduced in the smokers. Treadmill studies of 47 airmen showed that smokers had a decrease in respiratory minute volume and a lower oxygen consumption at equivalent heart rates than nonsmokers.[2]

SMOKING AND AIR POLLUTION

Many of the effects of inhaling cigarette smoke are similar to the effects of breathing highly polluted air. People install air conditioners in their homes and places of work, or travel out of the cities, to get away from polluted air. Yet, curiously, many of them continue voluntarily to inhale the most intensely polluted air to which man is exposed. The following excellent discussion, closely related to these facts and phenomena, was presented as an editorial in the highly respected magazine *Science* under the title "A Damaging Source of Air Pollution": [3]

Public concern about air pollution has grown rapidly during the past few years. In a recent poll, 80 percent of respondents felt that additional measures should be taken to minimize this problem. Most people, when they consider air pollution, think of the automobile, the smokestack, or the trash burner. Few

[2] Kenneth H. Cooper, George O. Guy, and R. A. Battenberg, "Effects of Cigarette Smoking on Endurance Performance," Journal of the American Medical Association, vol. 203, no. 3, p. 189, Jan. 15, 1968.
[3] Editorial by Philip H. Abelson in Science, vol. 158, Dec. 22, 1967. Reprinted with permission from the American Association for the Advancement of Science.

point to a most damaging source of air polution—the cigarette.

One of the toxic products of the automobile is carbon monoxide. Exposure for 1 hour to a concentration of this gas of 120 parts per million causes inactivation of about 5 percent of the body's hemoglobin and commonly leads to dizziness, headache, and lassitude. Concentrations of carbon monoxide as high as 100 ppm often occur in garages, in tunnels, and behind automobiles. Such concentrations are tiny in comparison with those (42,000 ppm) found in cigarette smoke. The smoker survives because most of the time he breathes air not so heavily polluted. However, in a poorly ventilated, smoke-filled room, concentrations of carbon monoxide can easily reach several hundred parts per million, thus exposing smokers and nonsmokers present to a toxic hazard.

Another air pollutant issuing from automobiles is nitrogen dioxide. Nitrogen dioxide is an acutely irritating gas; also, it gives rise to nitrite, a potential mutagenic agent. Concentrations of NO_2 as high as 3 ppm have been noted in Los Angeles, and levels of 5 ppm are considered dangerous. Cigarette smoke contains 250 parts of NO_2 per million.

Many of the toxic agents in cigarette smoke do not have counterparts in ordinary air pollution. One of these, hydrogen cyanide, is particularly noteworthy. It is highly active against respiratory enzymes. Long-term exposure to levels above 10 ppm is dangerous. The concentration in cigarette smoke is 1600 ppm.

These inorganic pollutants are three of many noxious substances that have been found in tobacco smoke. Among others are acrolein, aldehydes, phenols, and carcinogens, an important one of which is benzo(a)pyrene. Evidence points to synergistic effects among the toxic agents. The phenols, though not themselves notably carcinogenic, increase markedly the carcinogenic potency of benzpyrene.

The toxic effects of cigarette smoke are also enhanced by other environmental factors. A recent study of asbestos workers showed a very high incidence of lung cancer among smokers, in contrast to a low incidence among nonsmokers. In a group of 283 asbestos workers who had a history of cigarette smoking, 24 of 78 deaths were due to bronchogenic carcinoma. Of 87 asbestos workers who were nonsmokers, none died of lung cancer during a comparable period. A study of the uranium miners stricken with lung cancer has also revealed an effect related to smoking. The rate of fatalities was much higher among smokers than among nonsmokers.

Another example of a synergistic effect is seen in the smoker who breathes polluted urban air. The incidence of lung cancer among smokers is higher in the city than in rural areas.

The principal effects of smoking are borne by the smokers themselves. They pay for their habit with chronic disease and shortened life. Involved are the individual's decision and his life. However, when the individual smokes in a poorly ventilated space in the presence of others, he infringes the rights of others and becomes a serious contributor to air pollution.

TOBACCO & CANCER

Cancer is a condition in which certain cells of the body reproduce wildly and without limit. It is a disease, or rather a group of diseases, found in all ages and all races of man. Cancer was known to the early Egyptians many centuries ago, and the Romans, who were well acquainted with its appearance, observed how it extended into surrounding tissues. The Latin word "cancer" means "crab," and from its appearance the condition derived its name. The columns of cancer cells invading surrounding tissues resembled the appendages of a crab; the center of growth corresponded to the body of the crab.

The words "cancer" and "tumor" are not synonymous. A tumor, or neoplasm (new growth), is an overgrowth of tissue which serves no useful purpose. Tumors may be benign or malignant. Benign tumors do not spread to distant parts of the body, and unless they

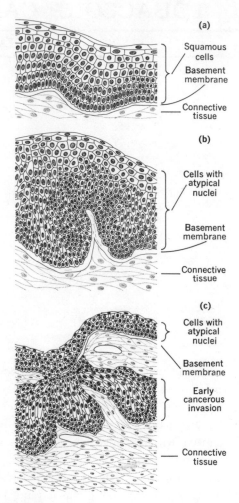

(a)

Squamous
cells
Basement
membrane

Connective
tissue

(b)

Cells with
atypical
nuclei

Basement
membrane

Connective
tissue

(c)

Cells with
atypical
nuclei

Basement
membrane

Early
cancerous
invasion

Connective
tissue

Figure 6.1. *Microscopic sections of* (a) *normal skin,* (b) *abnormal cells appearing, and* (c) *cancer beginning to invade.* (*Courtesy American Cancer Society.*)

cause pressure on vital organs, they are not generally dangerous to life. Malignant tumors, or cancers, infiltrate the tissues, destroy them locally, and spread to distant organs through blood vessels and lymph channels. This process of colonization, as it might be

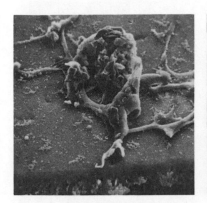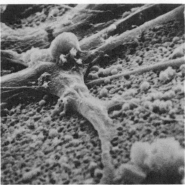

Figure 6.2. *Cancer cells in tissue culture.* Left: *a group of fibroblasts grow-ing on a fine millipore surface. The cells do not adhere and do not form compact colonies.* Right: *a fibroblast transformed with polyoma virus. This cell is able to spread and migrate on fine millipore. Magnification: 40,000X, through the stereoscan micro-scope. (Courtesy American Cancer Society. Source: Chester Beattie Research Institute, London, England.)*

designated, is known as *metastasis*, which comes from the Greek word meaning "standing after" or "placing in another way." Cancers may spread to nearby tissues directly as well as by metastasis.

THE CAUSES OF CANCER

Since there are many different types of cancer, most students of the disease believe that there are multiple causes, not one single cause. Some eminent scientists think that certain human cancers will eventually be proved to be due to or initiated by viruses, as is already known to be true for some cancers of animals and birds and for warts in man.

Whatever the cause or causes of cancer, the basic process is a change in the DNA or RNA, i.e., in the chemicals (or molecules)

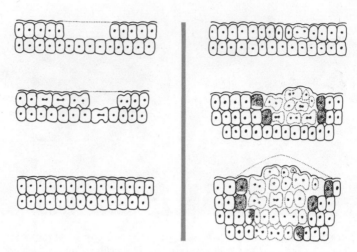

Figure 6.3. Left, top to bottom: *damaged body tissue (note area of missing cells) undergoing normal, orderly cell replacement, and healing.* Right, top to bottom: *injured area (note grayed cells) suffering from beginnings of abnormal, disorderly, malignant growth of cancer. (Source: American Cancer Society.)*

which constitute the reproductive mechanism, or genes, of a cell. As a result of this change the cell loses its normal reproductive restraint and begins to reproduce without limit. The cancer cell tends to be larger than the normal cell, and its nucleus is disproportionately large in relation to total cell size. In dividing, it may produce three or more new cells instead of two, as in normal cell division. The cancer cell is less adhesive to adjacent cells than are normal cells.

If a virus is the cause, it probably combines with and alters the genes of the cell, to make the cell cancerous. If chemical or metabolic disturbances are the cause, they too act through their effect upon the genes.

Even though the fundamental cause of cancer is a disturbance in the genes of cells, *contributory factors* are commonly spoken of as causes of cancer. Prominent among these are cigarette smoke in lung cancer; sunlight, soot, or other irritating substances in skin cancer; and radiation in leukemia and in cancer of the bones. Such contributory factors may be the trigger mechanisms that upset the balance between cancer viruses and body cells, or they may disturb the chemical processes of the cell in a manner that causes a similar result.

The most common form of cancer is called *carcinoma*. This arises in cells of the body surfaces such as the skin, lips, surface of the cervix, and in the linings of the mouth, larynx, trachea, bronchus, esophagus, stomach, rectum, colon, bladder, and uterus. The technical name for the type of lung cancer associated with smoking is *bronchogenic carcinoma*, meaning that it arises in the lining of the bronchial tubes through which air passes to various parts of the lungs. The principal types of bronchogenic carcinoma are called *epidermoid carcinoma*, *undifferentiated carcinoma*, and *adenocarcinoma*. The great majority of cases are of the first two types, both of which are highly related to cigarette smoking. The third type, adenocarcinoma, is far less common and less related to smoking.

Cancer (carcinoma) can be produced experimentally by applying certain chemicals, known as *carcinogens*, to tissues such as the skin of an animal. This is done by painting the skin repeatedly with some carcinogen such as 3-4 benzpyrene. Usually, such applications must take place for several months to produce cancer in short-lived animals like mice, rats, and guinea pigs. Many of these chemicals can cause cancer in human beings, but it usually takes years for cancer to develop because of the relatively low concentrations of these chemicals to which man may be exposed.

CANCER OF THE LUNG

The first report of a notable increase in lung cancer deaths based upon autopsy records was made by Dr. Moses Barron of the Uni-

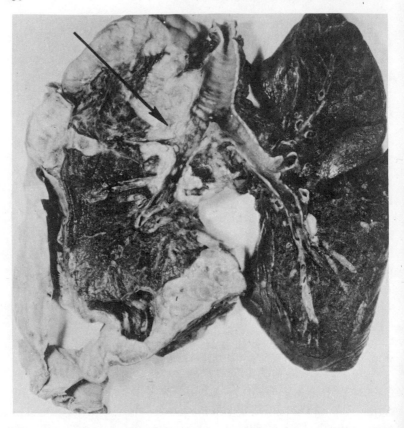

Figure 6.4. *The cancerous lung of a heavy smoker. Arrow indicates malignant area. (Courtesy American Cancer Society.)*

versity of Minnesota. In the period July 1, 1920, to June 20, 1921, Dr. Barron and his associates (of whom the author of this book was one) made a diagnosis of lung cancer at autopsy in eight persons. Lung cancer was then a very rare disease. In fact, Dr. Barron's review of autopsy records at the University over the twenty-year period 1899 to 1919 revealed only four cases of lung cancer. By contrast, in 1967 lung cancer was recorded, on University of Minnesota autopsy reports, as the cause of 92 deaths.

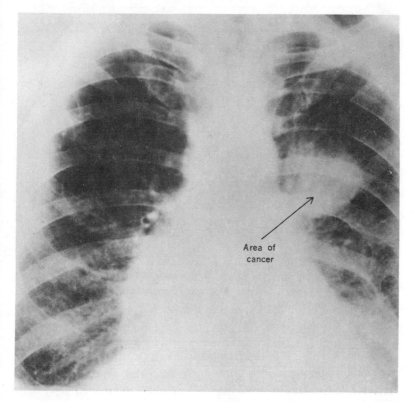

Area of
cancer

Figure 6.5. An X-ray of a cancerous lung. The shadowed area (arrow) indicates the presence of a tumor so large that surgery would
probably prove useless. (Courtesy American Cancer Society.)

Today cancer of the lung is the leading cause of cancer deaths in
this country. Its increase has been so rapid in recent years that it is
frequently referred to as an epidemic. In 1914 only 371 deaths in
the United States were reported as due to lung cancer. In 1930,
this number rose to 2,357; in 1940, to 7,121; in 1950, to 18,313; in
1960, to 36,420; and in 1968, to 55,300—46,600 deaths of men and
8,700 deaths of women. If present trends continue until the year
2000, there will be approximately 125,000 deaths annually from
lung cancer in this country.

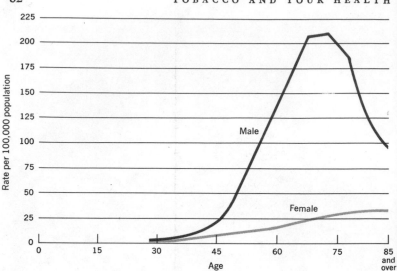

Figure 6.6. *Death rates for cancer of the lung, United States, 1965, by age and sex. (Source: American Cancer Society and U.S. Public Health Service.)*

As noted earlier, in both retrospective and prospective studies lung cancer stands out more prominently than any other disease in its relation to cigarette smoking. All studies of this subject have arrived at essentially identical conclusions. For an understanding of them it is necessary therefore to consider only the findings of the largest and most recent of these studies, the one which involved a follow-up of more than a million men and women for almost four years. (For an explanation of this study, see page 29.) This study shows that death rates increase in relation to the following factors:

    1 *The number of cigarettes smoked:* According to death certificates (on which 88 percent of the diagnoses were confirmed by reports from doctors and 65 to 70 percent by microscopic examination), the risk of dying from lung cancer for men aged 35 to 84 who smoke less than one pack of cigarettes a day is six times as great, and for men who smoke

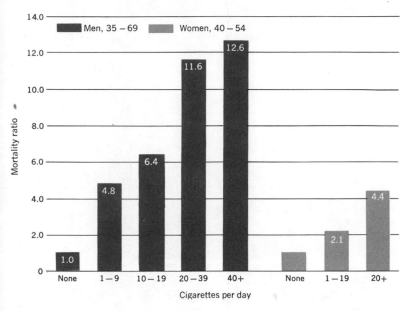

Figure 6.7. *Lung cancer deaths of men and women, in relation to number of cigarettes smoked per day. Diagnoses based on death certificates. (Source: American Cancer Society.)*

two or more packs a day sixteen times as great, as for non-smokers; for women who smoke a pack or more a day the risk of dying from lung cancer is more than four times as great as for women who do not smoke.

2 *Inhalation:* If one inhales, about 90 percent of the particulate matter (tar and nicotine) in the smoke is retained in the body; if one does not inhale, only about 10 percent. Everyone who smokes inhales some of the smoke, but the amount inhaled is very much greater for those who inhale consciously and purposefully.

Men who say that they do not inhale or inhale slightly have about eight times the risk and men who inhale deeply fourteen times the risk of lung cancer that nonsmokers have; the corresponding rates for women who do not inhale or

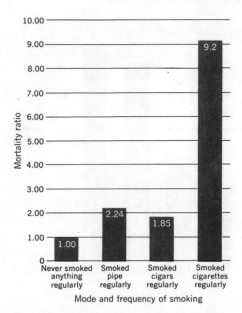

Figure 6.8. *Lung cancer in males, by type of smoking (age 35–84). (Source: American Cancer Society.)*

inhale slightly and for women who inhale moderately or deeply are 1.8 times and 3.7 times, respectively, the rates for women who do not smoke.

3 *Age of beginning to smoke:* Men who started smoking before 15 years of age run nearly five times as much risk of dying from lung cancer as men who started smoking after the age of 25; women who started smoking before age 25 run twice as much risk of dying from lung cancer as women who did not start smoking until after 25.

Two reasons for the greater risk for persons who start to smoke early in life are that the lungs are exposed to cigarette smoke for more years and that those who start smoking early in life in general inhale more and smoke more heavily than those who start smoking later in life. It is also possible that the lung tissue is particularly susceptible to the effects of cigarette smoke in early life.

THE DISCONTINUANCE OF SMOKING

Recent research indicates that if one stops smoking before cancer has actually started, lung tissue tends to repair itself, even if so-called precancerous changes are present. The beneficial effects of giving up smoking even for those who have smoked for years are obvious from Figure 4.5. Beginning one year after the cessation of smoking, the risk of lung cancer decreases progressively, until after ten years it is only slightly higher than for those who have never been regular smokers.

LUNG CANCER IN NONSMOKERS

Although lung cancer can and sometimes does develop in non-smokers, the rarity of this is indicated by the conclusion of Dr. Brian MacMahon, professor of epidemiology at the Harvard School of Public Health, that at least 90 percent of lung cancer deaths would not occur if people did not smoke cigarettes.

AIR POLLUTION AND LUNG CANCER

As noted in the previous chapter, tobacco smoke is the most intensely polluted air breathed. If the general atmosphere were as heavily polluted as tobacco smoke, it would be impossible to see across the street. Furthermore, the smoke from a cigarette, pipe, or cigar is taken directly into the mouth, throat, and respiratory tract, thereby bypassing the filtration mechanism of the nose which normally removes at least 75 percent of the foreign matter from the air.

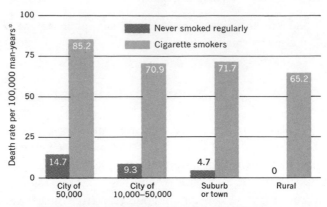

*Man-years = number of men observed, multiplied by number of
years over which the observations were made.

Figure 6.9. *Air pollution and lung cancer; death rates in urban and rural
areas: nonsmokers and cigarette smokers.* (*Source: Hammond
and Horn,* Journal of the American Medical Association, *vol.
166, pp. 1159, 1295, 1958.*)

To most people, however, air pollution means general pollution of
the atmosphere. This is understandable and appropriate because
the air we breathe is polluted by smoke, soot, chemicals, and the
fumes from the combustion of gasoline and fuel oil. These air
pollutants contain substances known to be carcinogenic or cancer-
producing, as well as substances that cause chronic bronchitis and
emphysema. (See pages 87–95.)

Studies show that city dwellers have more lung cancer than country dwellers. The difference, however, is small compared with the
greatly increased death rates of cigarette smokers whether they live
in the country, in towns, or in cities. In Iceland, a region having
essentially no air pollution, cigarette smoking was unpopular and
lung cancer was rare prior to 1940. During the Second World War
Icelanders took up smoking, and the lung cancer death rate in
1951–1959 was five times that of 1930–1940. Commenting on
this change, Dr. Neils Dungal of the University of Iceland reports
that "the city of Reykjavik where most of the lung cancer occurs
has the purest air in Europe."

Studies in California show that for *nonsmokers* the death rate from lung cancer is a little higher in Los Angeles, a severe smog area, than in areas of the state with little or no air pollution. Among cigarette smokers, however, the death rate in cities with air pollution like Los Angeles is vastly greater. This strongly suggests that cigarette smoking and urban air pollution act *together* to cause a higher incidence of lung cancer than the sum of the two independently would cause.

In spite of the evidence of a very minimal relationship between lung cancer and general air pollution, many people believe that air pollution is a major cause of lung cancer. This misconception is due largely to the extensive publicity given by the tobacco industry's public relations firms to any statements that suggest a possible relationship of air pollution to cancer.

LUNG CANCER IN ASBESTOS WORKERS AND URANIUM MINERS

It has been known for some time that the continued inhalation of asbestos dust results in an increase in fibrous tissue in the lungs and the disease *asbestosis*. In addition, studies have shown that asbestos workers die of lung cancer at a rate 7 or 8 times as high as the general population. However, the risk of dying from lung cancer for asbestos workers who smoke cigarettes is 92 times as great as for nonsmokers of the same age in the general population. This indicates that while exposure to asbestos dust involves a risk of lung cancer, this risk is greatly increased by a combination of asbestos exposure with cigarette smoking.

Uranium miners also have been known to have high death rates from lung cancer. Recent studies, however, have shown that among uranium miners who do not smoke lung cancer is little if any more frequent than among nonsmokers in other occupations.

In fact, the U.S. Public Health Service has reported that out of 101 cases of lung cancer in uranium miners 100 were cigarette smokers; also that lung cancer is practically nonexistent among Indian uranium miners, most of whom rarely smoke. Here again cigarette smoke and dust from occupational exposure seem to act together to greatly increase the lung cancer hazard.

DIAGNOSIS AND TREATMENT

The most common symptoms that bring persons with lung cancer to physicians are chronic cough, blood-streaked sputum, chest pain, and shortness of breath. Unfortunately, by the time these symptoms appear the disease is usually advanced.

Occasionally, lung cancer is diagnosed early in connection with routine physical examinations or as a result of the chest x-rays recommended every six, or better every three, months for regular cigarette smokers. The microscopic examination of the sputum of smokers is useful as an aid in the recognition of the early development of lung cancer.

The most effective treatment of lung cancer is surgical removal of the diseased lung. When this was done before cancer cells had spread to other tissues, some hospitals report that 30 to 35 percent of patients have survived up to five years or more. Overall, however, only about 5 percent of patients with lung cancer survive five years after diagnosis.

X-ray treatment and/or treatment with special drugs are used in patients for whom surgical removal of the cancer is impossible. These therapies may also be used to destroy cancer cells that may have remained after surgery. In patients in whom the cancer has not been removed, these treatments frequently slow the progress of the disease but *very rarely* result in a cure.

ORAL CANCER

A century ago, Bouisson reported a convincing relationship between the use of tobacco and cancers of the oral cavity. (See page 16.) A few years ago it was observed that some carcinogenic substances in tobacco smoke fluoresce under ultraviolet light. A microscopic examination under ultraviolet light was therefore made of tissues of the mouths of smokers and nonsmokers. The study showed that when a person smokes tobacco, fluorescent material penetrates the cells of the lining of the mouth. In other words, material from tobacco smoke actually enters these cells.

Cancers of the lip, tongue, pharynx, and other tissues inside the mouth occur with greatly increased frequency in persons who smoke, chew tobacco, or use snuff. Dr. George Moore of the Roswell Park Memorial Institute of Buffalo, New York, reported that of 40 men with cancer of the mouth, 26 chewed tobacco or used snuff, and of 23 men with leukoplakia, there were 18 men who chewed tobacco or used snuff.

Hammond found the death rate from cancers of the tissues of the oral cavity ten times as high in cigarette smokers and five times as high in pipe and cigar smokers as in nonsmokers.

Snuff, particularly when used in the form of a pellet and held for long periods of time between the gum and the cheek, frequently causes irritation and eventually produces cancer at the spot. Such cancers, which may involve the bones of the jaw and face, are very common in India where it is a frequent practice to mix tobacco and a ground-up betel nut, wrap the mixture in a lemon leaf, and hold it for hours in the mouth. In South India this author saw large hospital wards filled with patients who had advanced cancers of this type.

OTHER CANCERS
ASSOCIATED
WITH SMOKING

Cancer of the larynx is 6 times as frequent and cancer of the esophagus 4 times as frequent in male cigarette smokers 45 to 64 years of age as in nonsmokers. Similar rates for other cancers are as follows: cancer of the pancreas 2.7 times as high in cigarette smokers as in nonsmokers; cancer of the liver and biliary passages 2.8 times as high; cancer of the urinary bladder 2 times as high; cancer of the stomach and the kidney, and leukemia 1.4 times as high.

Pipe and cigar smokers have rates for cancer of the lung 2 times as high as nonsmokers; for cancer of the buccal cavity 4.9 times as high; for cancer of the esophagus and cancer of the larynx 3 to 4 times as high.

Women smokers have death rates 2.2 times as high as nonsmokers for lung cancer; 1.8 times as high for cancer of the mouth, larynx, esophagus, and pancreas. The rate of increase of these cancers among women, however, has become as rapid as among men. And in view of the great increase in smoking by women in recent years, future death rates for cancers associated with smoking may well catch up with the rates for men.

PATHOLOGIC EVIDENCE

Extensive microscopic studies have been made of tissues lining the bronchial tubes of men and women who died of various causes. The findings may be summarized briefly as follows:

When people die of lung cancer, additional tiny cancers can some-times be found if the entire lungs are examined microscopically. In other words, lung cancer victims occasionally have two or more separate cancers in their bronchial tubes. In addition, they have numerous carcinomas *in situ*, i.e., cancers which have not invaded underlying tissues. The cells of a carcinoma *in situ* appear to be similar to the cells in the main mass of cancer which killed the patient. Similar cells, the nuclei of which look like the nuclei of cancer cells, are found widely scattered throughout the lining of the bronchial tubes of these patients.

Similar studies have been made of the lungs of men and women who died of causes other than lung cancer. Cell changes charac-teristic of carcinoma *in situ* rarely are found in the bronchial tubes of people who never smoked. On the other hand, many such changes occur in the lungs of cigarette smokers. Moreover, the number of abnormal cells increases with the amount of cigarette smoking. The linings of the bronchial tubes of most heavy ciga-rette smokers who died of causes other than lung cancer closely resemble those of persons who died of lung cancer. That is, they contain what appear to be carcinomas *in situ* as well as many cells with nuclei identical in appearance to the nuclei of cancer cells.

The bronchial tubes of cigar and pipe smokers usually show some similar changes but less change than those of cigarette smokers.

Among cigarette smokers, the number of cells resembling cancer cells increases with age, i.e., with the number of years of exposure to cigarette smoke. Few if any such cells are found in the bronchial tubes of nonsmokers, and there is no evidence of increase with advancing age.

Recent studies by Drs. Auerbach and Hammond and their asso-ciates have shown abnormal and apparently precancerous cells in the lungs of dogs that have been taught to smoke cigarettes through a tube inserted into the trachea. In the experiment reported, five dogs smoked up to six cigarettes every morning and afternoon for 421 days. A much longer period of time is necessary for the development of invasive cancer.[1]

Another recent study reports for the first time the development of cancer of the lung in mice from breathing a cigarette smoke and air mixture. Exposure of the mice was 12 minutes every other day for the greater part of their lives. The authors commented that the number of tumors might have been greater if the mice had been exposed more frequently to the smoke; for example, twice a day instead of once every two days.

The cancers reported are similar to the lung cancers in man caused by cigarette smoking. Futhermore mice which had been exposed to cigarette smoke for a long time developed emphysema. Very important also is the high death rate which occurred among the mice with even this small exposure to cigarette smoke.[2]

Briefly summarized, the evidence that cigarette smoking causes lung cancer is (1) cigarette smoke contains substances that produce cancer in animals; (2) lung cancer and several other cancers are many times more frequent among cigarette smokers than among nonsmokers; (3) the incidence of these cancers increases with the amount of smoking, the duration of smoking, and the degree of inhalation, and decreases with the cessation of smoking.

[1] Oscar Auerbach, E. C. Hammond, David Kirman, Lawrence Garfinkel, and Arthur Purdy Stout, ''Histologic Changes in Bronchial Tubes of Cigarette-smoking Dogs,'' Cancer, vol. 20, p. 2055, December, 1967.
[2] R. J. C. Harris and G. Negroni, ''Production of Lung Carcinomas in C57BL Mice Exposed to a Cigarette Smoke and Air Mixture,'' British Medical Journal, December, 1967, p. 637.

TOBACCO &
CARDIOVASCULAR DISEASE

Buerger's disease, a rare but serious disease of the blood vessels, has long been recognized as due primarily to the use of tobacco. (See page 19.) In this disease, which is also called *thromboangiitis obliterans*, blood flow to the extremities is progressively reduced. In advanced cases, gangrene, particularly of the lower extremities, frequently occurs and amputation of the affected part—toes, fingers, legs, or arms—becomes necessary. Patients with Buerger's disease must discontinue completely the use of tobacco in any form. If this is not done or if smoking is resumed, the disease is reactivated and may result in further gangrene and amputations. That this sometimes occurs is convincing evidence of the addictive power of tobacco.

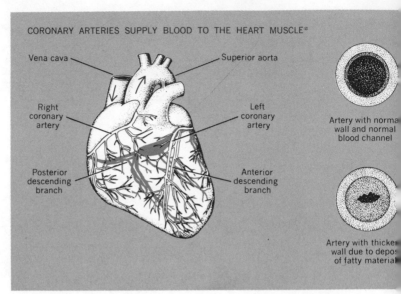

CORONARY ARTERIES SUPPLY BLOOD TO THE HEART MUSCLE*

Vena cava

Superior aorta

Right coronary artery

Left coronary artery

Posterior descending branch

Anterior descending branch

Artery with normal wall and normal blood channel

Artery with thicker wall due to deposit of fatty material

*Clots in narrowed, irregular portions of the coronary arteries are likely to result in heart attacks.

Figure 7.1. *Coronary arteries, thrombosis, and infarction.*

CORONARY HEART DISEASE

The most frequent cause of death in this country is coronary heart disease, also called *coronary thrombosis* or *myocardial infarction*. Numerous studies over the past fifteen or twenty years have shown a definite association between this disease and cigarette smoking. Coronary heart disease occurs when a coronary artery or one of its branches becomes plugged or obstructed. The plugging is usually due to the formation of a thrombus (clot) within the artery. Since the coronary arteries provide the heart muscle with blood, the portion of the heart muscle supplied by the artery in which a thrombus occurs loses its source of oxygen and food and so dies. Such an area of heart muscle is called an *infarct*, and the condition myocardial infarction. (Figure 7.2.) If one of the larger branches of a coronary artery becomes plugged, the shock to the heart may be so great that it stops contracting or beating effectively and sudden death results.

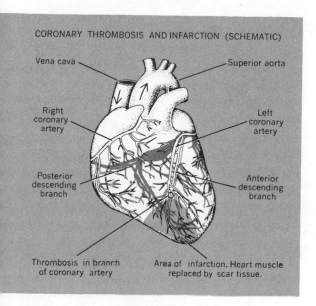

CORONARY THROMBOSIS AND INFARCTION (SCHEMATIC)

Vena cava

Superior aorta

Right coronary artery

Left coronary artery

Posterior descending branch

Anterior descending branch

Thrombosis in branch of coronary artery

Area of infarction. Heart muscle replaced by scar tissue.

Coronary thrombosis is the most common cause of death from heart disease. However, between 60 and 70 percent of those stricken survive the first attack. When this occurs, the necrotic (dead) muscle in the area of infarction is replaced by scar tissue, but usually enough functioning heart muscle remains to meet the body's needs. Subsequent attacks are likely to occur, but these may be delayed many years during which the individual is able to live a relatively normal life.

An obstruction, partial or complete, of the coronary arteries is frequently accompanied by severe attacks of pain, called *angina pectoris*. This pain usually originates in the region of the heart and radiates to the left shoulder and down the left arm.

Coronary thombosis is much more serious in young persons than in older persons. Younger victims are frequently individuals who have been active, even physically powerful, but, for various reasons, have slipped into a kind of muscular retirement. It seems

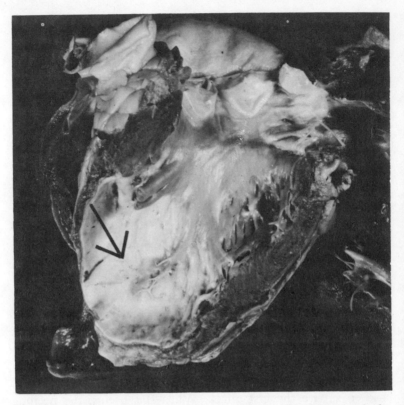

Figure 7.2. *Heart with area of infarction. (Courtesy Dr. Oscar Auerbach.)*

that sedentary living predisposes people to coronary heart disease and that regular, moderate physical activity lessens its likelihood. This holds true for individuals who have had coronary thrombosis and infarction as well as for those who have never had heart trouble.

In 1940 a study of 2,400 electrocardiograms of healthy males showed 50 percent more abnormal tracings of smokers than of non-smokers.[1] This was suggestive of heart damage, but the asso-

---

[1] H. J. Johnson, "A Study of 2400 Electrocardiograms of Apparently Healthy Males," Journal American Medical Association, vol. 114, p. 561, Feb. 16, 1940.

ciation of cigarette smoking and coronary heart disease was first convincingly demonstrated by the prospective studies of smokers and nonsmokers described in Chapter 4. The most recent study of this type, conducted by Dr. E. Cuyler Hammond, involved a million men and women and resulted in the following conclusions: [2]

1 Death rates from coronary heart disease for men and women 45 to 54 years of age are 2.8 times as high for men and 2 times as high for women who smoke a package or more of cigarettes a day as for nonsmokers.

2 Death rates increase with the number of cigarettes smoked per day, with the degree of inhalation, and with the age at which smoking was begun—it is one-third higher for those who started to smoke before 15 than for those who started after 25 years of age.

3 The greatest relative risk of death from heart disease among smokers as compared with nonsmokers is in the age group 40 to 49, with less difference in each succeeding decade.

4 Coronary death rates are little higher for pipe and cigar smokers than for nonsmokers.

5 Death rates decrease with the cessation of smoking.

6 Microscopic examinations of the hearts of persons who are killed or who die from diseases other than coronary heart disease show that there are more plaques—that is, raised, roughened spots upon which thrombi tend to develop—and much more extensive atherosclerosis in the coronary arteries of smokers than of nonsmokers. (See Figure 7.5.)

The American Heart Association, in testimony before the U.S. Senate Commerce Committee in 1965, stated that about 125,000 preventable deaths from cardiovascular disease in the United States each year are associated with cigarette smoking.

[2] E. C. Hammond, "Smoking in Relation to the Death Rates of One Million Men and Women," National Cancer Institute, Monograph 19, Jan., 1966, pp. 127–204.

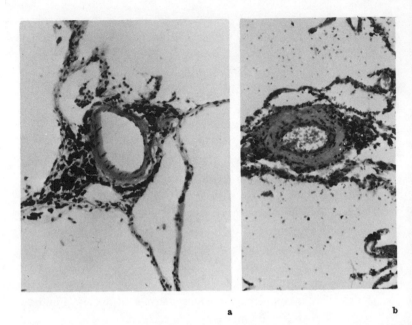

a   b

Figure 7.3. *Continual cigarette smoking makes the walls of a normal artery
(a) thicken until they almost touch (b, c, d) and close off the
vital passageway. (Courtesy Dr. Oscar Auerbach.)*

Many more deaths from heart disease than from lung cancer are
attributable to smoking; yet most people know that cigarette
smoking is associated with lung cancer, but relatively few realize its
association with heart disease. The major reasons for this are:

    1   The association of cigarette smoking with lung cancer was
well established before its association with heart disease was
recognized.

    2   Cigarette smoking is responsible for most of the deaths from
lung cancer, while such factors as high blood pressure, increased amounts of cholesterol in the blood, overweight, and
lack of exercise contribute to coronary heart disease.

    3   The risk of a heavy smoker dying from lung cancer is approxi-
mately twenty times that of a nonsmoker, while the risk of a

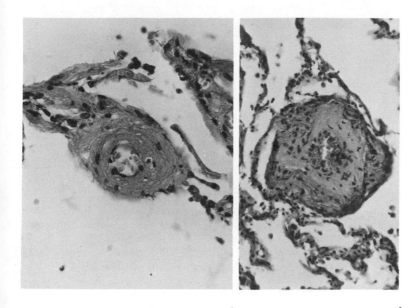

c   d

heavy smoker dying from coronary heart disease is about three times that of a nonsmoker. However, there are so many more deaths from coronary heart disease than from lung cancer (559,293 versus 48,433 in 1965) that the total number of deaths from coronary disease attributable to smoking is two and a half to three times the number of deaths from lung cancer caused by smoking.

According to Professor Hardin Jones of the University of California, the mortality curve of coronary heart disease for individuals who smoke one pack per day is shifted by seven years from the curve for nonsmokers. That is, the probability that a cigarette smoker will die of coronary heart disease at age 55 is the same as

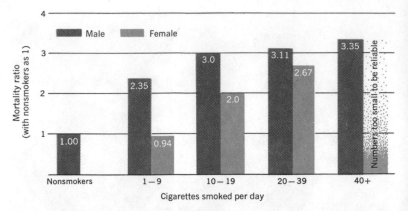

Figure 7.4. Coronary heart disease and cigarette smoking: mortality ratios of men and women (age 45–54), by number of cigarettes smoked per day. (Source: E. C. Hammond, Smoking in Relation to the Death Rates of One Million Men and Women, National Cancer Institute monograph No. 19, pp. 146–147, 1966.)

the probability that a nonsmoker will die of coronary heart disease at age 62. With respect to coronary heart disease, then, the cigarette smoker behaves as though his physiological age was seven years greater than his chronological age.

Significant also is the fact that the greatest relative risk of dying from coronary heart disease associated with cigarette smoking is in the age group 40 to 50. This is almost twenty years earlier than the age of greatest risk of dying from lung cancer caused by smoking.

A study by the Health Insurance Plan of Greater New York involving some 110,000 adult men and women reveals that male smokers as a whole are twice as likely to suffer heart attacks as nonsmokers and that smokers who are physically inactive are three times as likely to suffer attacks as smokers who have been physically active. Also, if a smoker has a heart attack, his chances of surviving are twice as good if he has been physically active. The study concludes that to avoid heart attacks it is best to be a non-smoker who is at least moderately active. Such an individual is

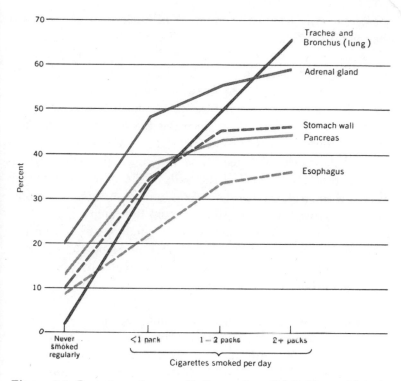

Figure 7.5. *Percentage of men with "more than slight" fibrous thickening of walls of arterioles, by smoking habits. Figures are standardized for age. (Source: Auerbach, Hammond, and Garfinkel.)*

nine times less likely to have a fatal heart attack than his inactive smoking counterpart.[3]

REASONS FOR ASSOCIATION OF HEART DISEASE AND SMOKING

The reasons for the association of smoking and coronary heart disease are not completely understood. However, studies show that

[3] Charles W. Frank et al., "Myocardial Infarction in Men: Role of Physical Activity and Smoking in Incidence and Mortality," Journal of the American Medical Association, vol. 198, p. 1241, Dec. 19, 1966.

smokers usually have larger amounts of cholesterol in the blood than nonsmokers; and it has been well established that high levels of cholesterol in the blood increase the risk of coronary heart disease. It has been shown also that for persons with high blood cholesterol the risk of coronary heart disease is increased by smoking. Other studies show that cigarette smoking accelerates the clotting of blood. This in turn increases the risk of the formation of clots—thrombi—in the coronary arteries. Pathological examinations of the hearts of humans and experimental studies of dogs show increased thickening of the walls of the arterioles and small arteries with smoking. This has been found in the lung, the esophagus, the stomach wall, the pancreas, and the adrenal glands. The degree of thickening increases with the amount of smoking and with age. To maintain an adequate flow of blood through such arteries and arterioles requires increased work by the heart.[4] (See Figure 7.3.)

The carbon monoxide in cigarette smoke (see page 41) reduces the oxygen-carrying capacity of the blood. Because of this the blood must be circulated more rapidly in order to provide the cells of the body with the oxygen which they require. This also throws an extra work load on the heart.

Investigators at the University of Copenhagen report that in their judgment carbon monoxide and cigarette smoking are more to blame than food habits for accelerating the arteriosclerotic process, now a factor in half of all deaths in Denmark.

Still another effect of smoking is fibrosis and loss of elasticity of the lungs (see page 87). This condition makes it more difficult for the heart to pump the blood through the lungs and, like the other factors mentioned above, may contribute to heart failure.

[4] Oscar Auerbach, E. C. Hammond, and Lawrence Garfinkel, "Thickening of Walls of Arterioles and Small Arteries in Relation to Age and to Smoking Habits," New England Journal of Medicine, vol. 278, p. 980, May 2, 1968.

CESSATION OF SMOKING
AND HEART DISEASE

Some people who stop smoking gain weight. Overweight is associated with an increased risk of heart disease. Therefore, it is argued—particularly by smokers who want an excuse to continue smoking—that any reduction in risk of coronary heart disease from giving up smoking is offset by the increased risk from overweight. That this is not true is evident from the fact that overall death rates of smokers from coronary heart disease decrease rapidly with the cessation of smoking. Thus the increased risk of coronary disease from the gain in weight that some smokers experience when they stop smoking is insignificant in comparison with the reduced risk which results from stopping smoking. In fact, it has been calculated that a man of average weight who smoked two packs of cigarettes a day would have to gain at least 75 pounds to offset the improvement in his life expectancy from stopping smoking.

CONCLUSIVE PROOF?

Some say, as did the author of a recent article, that it has not been conclusively proved that cigarette smoking causes coronary heart disease.[5] This is contrary to the opinion of the American Heart Association and every group that has studied this question. The evidence is overwhelming that cigarette smoking is consistently associated with coronary disease and that the risk of the disease increases with the amount of smoking and decreases with the cessation of smoking. Therefore, the only assumption that a responsible physician, health official, or individual can accept as a basis for a course of action is that the association is one of cause

[5] C. C. Seltzer, "An Evaluation of the Effect of Smoking on Coronary Heart Disease," Journal of the American Medical Association, vol. 203, pp. 193–200, 1968.

and effect—at least *until* it is proved otherwise and some other acceptable explanation is given for the association.

AORTIC ANEURYSM

Aortic aneurysm, a ballooning of the aorta due to a weakening of its walls, is significantly associated with cigarette smoking. When this condition develops, death usually follows rupture of the aneurysm. Why this disease occurs with increased frequency in cigarette smokers is unknown. Yet all surveys have confirmed this relationship. Hammond's recent study showed it to be 2.6 times as frequent as a cause of death among male smokers 45 to 64 and 3.9 times as frequent among women smokers as among nonsmokers. In heavy smokers these ratios are still higher.

STROKES

Stroke, also called *apoplexy*, produces sudden paralysis, usually with total or partial loss of consciousness and sensation. The cause may be the breaking of a blood vessel of the brain or an obstruction in such a vessel. If a blood vessel breaks, the resulting hemorrhage causes pressure on the cells of the brain, with impairment of blood flow and brain damage. Obstruction due to a thrombus (clot) or to an embolus impedes or prevents the flow of blood to the portions of the brain served by the artery in which the obstruction occurs. In either case, if the brain cells do not receive sufficient oxygen, permanent damage will result.

Strokes cause the death of more than 200,000 Americans a year. Of these, 80 percent are people aged 65 and over. Thus, strokes more than coronary heart disease or cancer affect primarily the aged. In young persons strokes are less likely to be fatal, but in many instances they are more tragic because of the years of disability which result. It is estimated that almost two million people now alive in the United States have suffered major strokes. Many more have had minor strokes, some diagnosed and many unrecognized.

For many victims of stroke the resulting disability is a tragedy worse than death. Some fight their way back through willpower and determination. Goya, at forty-six, had a stroke, becoming deaf and losing the use of his hands. He fought back and gradually learned to make his hands work, going on to paint some of his greatest works of art later in his life. Louis Pasteur also suffered a stroke at the age of forty-six. His left leg was permanently paralyzed and the use of his left arm and hand greatly impaired. Yet he returned to work in his laboratory and carried out the research on the control of communicable disease which placed him everlastingly among the great men of science. Today many who have had strokes can be helped by rehabilitation programs which, if started early and carried through, can make the difference between total dependency and self-sufficiency.

The American Cancer Society study found that death rates from strokes are 74 percent higher among women and 38 percent higher among men who smoke cigarettes than among non-smokers; the greatest relative risk of death from strokes in people who smoke is in the surprisingly young age group 45 to 54. Paffenberger's follow-up study of Harvard graduates showed that those who smoked more than 10 cigarettes a day had twice as many strokes as those who smoked fewer cigarettes or none at all.

TOBACCO &
CHRONIC BRONCHITIS,
EMPHYSEMA, &
CERTAIN OTHER DISEASES

CHAPTER EIGHT

Chronic bronchitis is a persistent or recurrent inflammation of the bronchial tubes. Irritation of the cells lining the bronchial tubes causes the secretion of an excessive amount of mucus. This is followed by a chronic cough to expel the irritating material and the mucus. Persistent deep coughing and thick mucus make breathing increasingly difficult.

Emphysema, frequently associated with chronic bronchitis, is a disease in which the lungs lose their elasticity and cannot expand and contract normally to draw in and force out air. As the disease progresses, the walls of the alveoli, or air sacs, are gradually destroyed (Figures 8.2 to 8.4). The result is a slowly progressive, crippling disease which seriously reduces the ability of the lungs to obtain oxygen and get rid of carbon dioxide. This makes it necessary for the heart to work harder to maintain a flow of blood

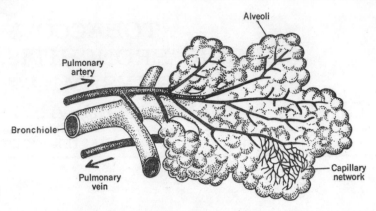

Figure 8.1. *Bronchioles, alveoli, and blood vessels of lung. (Source: E. Cuyler Hammond, "The Effects of Smoking," Scientific American, July, 1962.)*

through the lungs and throughout the body sufficient to provide the cells, tissues, and organs with enough oxygen to meet their needs. The most common immediate cause of death from emphysema is heart failure.

Persistent cough, with or without expectoration, is the most common early symptom both of chronic bronchitis and of emphysema. This is frequently ignored or dismissed as "merely a cigarette cough." The most frequent reasons that these patients seek medical care are fatigue and shortness of breath. These symptoms may develop gradually, sometimes without significant cough. Unfortunately, by the time these patients see a physician more than half the lung tissue may have been destroyed. Lung tissue which has been destroyed does not regenerate. These patients, therefore, have to live the rest of their lives as partial or complete pulmonary cripples.

Deaths from chronic bronchitis and emphysema have increased from 2,038 in 1945 to 22,686 in 1965—a more rapid rise than has occurred for any other cause of death. At this rate of increase,

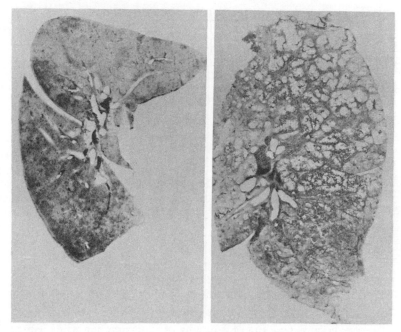

Figure 8.2. *Lung tissue. Left: normal lung tissue. Air sacs are too fine to be visible. Right: in emphysema, the lung tissue of a heavy smoker shows an abundance of greatly enlarged air sacs. Holes are areas of destroyed tissue. (Courtesy Dr. Oscar Auerbach.)*

100,000 persons in the United States will die from these diseases in 1975. If the effects of smoking on the lungs (Figures 8.2 and 8.3) were to be seen on the skin, few if any people would smoke.

Even more ominous is the rising toll of sickness and disability from these diseases. Patients with coronary heart disease or lung cancer usually recover or die in a relatively short time. Patients with chronic bronchitis and emphysema are partially or completely disabled for many years. Said a physician discussing a paper on lung cancer and smoking at the American Medical Association:

> I am a chest specialist. I make my living taking care of patients with chest diseases. I agree with everything that has

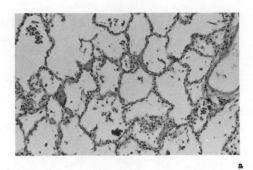

a

Figure 8.3. *Effect of cigarette smoking on microscopic appearance of alveolar walls:* (a) *normal lung tissue;* (b) *lung with emphysema;* (c) *lung with advanced emphysema.* (*Courtesy Dr. Oscar Auerbach.*)

been said about the seriousness of lung cancer, but I want to add that the person who gets lung cancer from smoking is lucky in comparison to the person who gets emphysema, because lung cancer is usually of short duration while patients with emphysema spend years of their lives gasping and struggling for breath.

My own roommate and closest friend in medical school did just this. Always a heavy cigarette smoker, he developed emphysema in his early fifties. It became necessary for him first to reduce and then to discontinue his medical practice. The last five years of his life were spent at home or in the hospital, most of the time with an oxygen tent by his side.

Emphysema incapacitates 1 out of 14 wage earners over 45. Over a million people in this country lead restricted lives because of emphysema. The Social Security Administration pays out in excess of $90 million a year to persons disabled by emphysema or chronic bronchitis. About 14,000 new victims of these diseases become Social Security claimants each year. In 1967 the U.S. Veterans

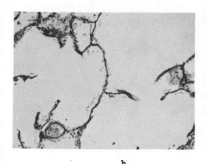
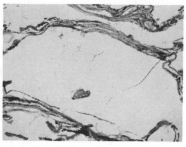

b   c

Administration doubled the number of its Medical Units for the treatment of emphysema, making a total of 52 such units in Veterans Administration hospitals.

CAUSES OF CHRONIC BRONCHITIS AND EMPHYSEMA

The causes of these diseases are multiple and include chronic irritation, repeated or chronic infections, bronchial asthma, and injury from coughing. The most plausible explanation, however, for the rapid increase in these chronic pulmonary diseases is the presence of new irritating inhalants not common before this century. General air pollution is one of these irritants, but cigarette smoking is of vastly greater importance. (See Table 8.1.) In fact, smoking produces the most intensely polluted air one breathes. (See page 52.)

In a ten-year study of British physicians the death rate for bronchitis and emphysema was 6.8 times as high for those who smoked 1 to 14 cigarettes a day as for physicians who did not smoke; 12.8

times as high for those who smoked 15 to 24 cigarettes a day; and
21.2 times as high for those who smoked 25 or more cigarettes a
day.[1]

In Dr. Hammond's study of a million men and women the death
rate for bronchitis and emphysema for men aged 45 to 64 was 6.6
times as high for those who smoked cigarettes as for nonsmokers;
in the age group 65 to 84 the corresponding rate was 11.4 times as
high. For women the rate was 4.9 times as high for all smokers as
for nonsmokers and 7.4 times as high for the "heavier smokers."
For pipe and cigar smokers the emphysema rate was 1.4 times as
high as for nonsmokers.[2]

TABLE 8.1 **Presence of bronchitis and of irreversible obstructive
lung disease (bronchitis and emphysema) in men as
percentage of population in the age group**

Type of smoker	Chronic bronchitis, percent	Irreversible obstructive lung disease, percent	Amount of smoking, cigarettes per day	Percent of patients with bronchitis
Nonsmokers	13.8	7.3	Nonsmokers	15.0
Former smokers	11.9	7.2	Former	
Pipe and cigar	26.0	12.3	smokers	18.9
Cigarettes	40.3	24.9	Current smokers:	
			1 to 10	29.8
			11 to 20	34.2
			21 to 30	42.3
			31 to 40	61.1
			41+	75.3

SOURCE: D. O. Anderson and B. A. Ferris, Jr.: "Role of Tobacco Smoking in
the Causation of Chronic Respiratory Disease," New England Journal
of Medicine, vol. 267, p. 787, 1962.

[1] R. Doll and A. B. Hill, "Mortality in Relation to Smoking: 10 Year Observation
of British Doctors," British Medical Journal, vol. 1, p. 1460, June, 1964.
[2] E. C. Hammond, "Smoking in Relation to the Death Rates of One Million Men and
Women," National Cancer Institute, Monograph 19, Jan., 1966.

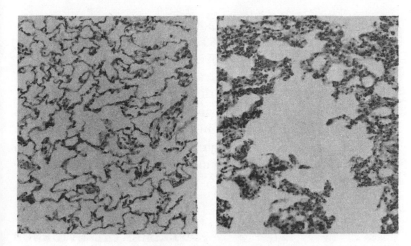

Figure 8.4. *Microscopic sections of dogs' lungs, showing tissue from* (left) *a nonsmoking, and* (right) *a smoking canine.* (*Right photo is more highly magnified.*) *The smoking animal had gone through 4,084 cigarettes in 423 days.* (Source: Oscar Auerbach, E. C. Hammond, David Kirman, and Lawrence Garfinkel, Journal of the American Medical Association, vol. 199, p. 241, January 23, 1967.

Dr. Edward A. Gaensler, Professor of Surgery at Boston University School of Medicine, predicts that emphysema will be responsible for the disability of about 20 million workers in five years' time. Most emphysema victims are men who die in their sixties. Since an increasing number of men of this age have been smoking for 30 to 40 years, we can anticipate a continuing increase in emphysema deaths. Among women the death rate from emphysema is currently much lower than among men. This is probably because few women in their sixties have smoked heavily and steadily since their teens. Since women now begin smoking as early as men, it is likely that emphysema will soon be a major cause of death in women as well. In fact, during the past 10 years, female deaths from emphysema have increased at the same rate as male deaths.

Dr. Roger S. Mitchell, distinguished specialist in diseases of the chest at the Webb-Waring Institute for Medical Research of the

University of Colorado, has reported that 95 percent of emphysema patients with a loss of 50 percent or more of their lung function are heavy cigarette smokers.

Studies also show that the death rate for chronic bronchitis and emphysema increases with the number of cigarettes smoked: less than a pack a day, five times as high as a nonsmoker; more than a pack a day, eight times as high. The degree of inhalation also increases the death rate but seems to be less important than the number of cigarettes smoked.

EXPERIMENTAL EVIDENCE

Many studies of the effects of cigarette smoke upon the trachea and bronchi of laboratory animals show that smoke first slows, then stops ciliary action and eventually destroys the cilia—the tiny hairlike structures whose protective functions were discussed on page 49. (See also Figure 5.7.)

In an experiment in which 10 dogs inhaled the smoke of up to 84 cigarettes a week, all developed various degrees of emphysema. This was undistinguishable microscopically from human emphysema.[3] Also, as we have noted, Dr. R. J. C. Harris of London reported emphysema in mice who inhaled a mixture of cigarette smoke and air (page 72).

In a large study thousands of sections of the lungs of smokers and nonsmokers who died from diseases not associated with smoking were examined microscopically. In these sections abnormal changes and thickening of the walls of the small branches of the bronchi and the alveoli were found regularly in smokers and very rarely in nonsmokers. In another study, 93 percent of smokers

[3] Oscar Auerbach, E. C. Hammond, David Kirman, and Lawrence Garfinkel, "Emphysema Produced in Dogs by Cigarette Smoking," Journal of the American Medical Association, vol. 199, p. 241, Jan. 23, 1967.

had abnormal cells in their lungs, but only 1.2 percent of non-smokers did.[4]

TREATMENT

Complete and immediate cessation of smoking is essential. This will reduce cough, expectoration, and other symptoms of bronchitis within a few weeks. Lung tissue which has been destroyed by emphysema is not replaced. Progress of the disease, however, is usually arrested or at least retarded by stopping smoking. Exposure to other irritants in the air and to respiratory infections should be avoided. A change of climate, particularly during the cold months, may be helpful. Medical treatments prescribed by physicians to meet the needs of individual patients are useful.

OTHER DISEASES ASSOCIATED WITH CIGARETTE SMOKING

Peptic ulcer This term includes ulcers of the stomach and the duodenum. Early studies suggested that smoking interferes with the healing of ulcers but drew no conclusions relative to causation. Subsequent studies indicate a strong relationship and one that must be considered causal until proved otherwise. Dr. Hammond's recent study showed that deaths from ulcers of the stomach are four times as frequent in smokers as in nonsmokers and deaths from ulcers of the duodenum three times as frequent.

Cirrhosis of the liver Cirrhosis of the liver is shown by several studies to be about twice as frequent a cause of death in cigarette

[4] O. Auerbach, A. P. Stout, E. C. Hammond, and L. Garfinkel, "Smoking Habits and Age in Relation to Pulmonary Changes, Rupture of Alveolar Septums and Thickening of Walls of Small Arteries and Arterioles," *New England Journal of Medicine*, vol. 26, p. 1045, Nov. 14, 1963.

smokers as in nonsmokers. However, since excessive use of alcohol contributes to cirrhosis of the liver and since most heavy drinkers are also heavy smokers, it is not clear whether cigarette smoking is independently related to cirrhosis of the liver.

EFFECTS OF SMOKING DURING PREGNANCY

In a study of 7,500 patients, the incidence of abortion and premature births was nearly twice as great for smoking mothers as for nonsmoking mothers; and the average weight of newborn infants of mothers who smoked regularly throughout pregnancy was 170 grams less than the weight of infants of mothers who never smoked. It is possible also that nursing infants may be affected by the traces of nicotine in the milk of mothers who smoke. Subsequent to the first printing of this book Dr. Jo Ann Haberman, Assistant Professor of Radiology at Temple University in Philadelphia, reported a study which shows visually that the smoking of a single cigarette reduces the blood flow not only to the fingers and toes but also to the placenta in the uterus of pregnant women. This means that a woman who smokes during pregnancy reduces the oxygen and the food supply to her unborn baby.

SMOKING AND LOSS OF TEETH

A study at Roswell Park Memorial Institute has shown that periodontal disease, particularly inflammation of the gums, destruction of supporting bony tissue, and loss of teeth, is much more frequent among smokers than among nonsmokers. It has also shown that women smokers between 20 and 39 years of age have twice as great a chance of developing advanced periodontal disease, and of losing some or all of their teeth, as have nonsmoking women in that age group. Further, the study indicates that men of any given age who smoke cigarettes develop as much periodontal disease as do nonsmoking men 15 years older; and that the chances of being toothless between 30 and 59 years of age are twice as great for men who smoke as for those who do not.[5]

SMOKING AND ACCIDENTS

Smoking contributes directly to accidents by causing fires. In 1965, 163,000 fires resulting in a property loss of $80 million were linked to smoking or to matches used in smoking. Although no complete record is available, it is estimated that about 1,800 people a year die from fires caused by smoking.

Several studies indicate a relation between smoking and traffic accidents. One such study from Columbia University reports that automobile accidents are four times as frequent for drivers who smoke cigarettes as for drivers who do not smoke. Similar relationships have been reported for industrial accidents. While the evidence is not sufficient to conclude that there is a cause-and-effect relationship, a report from the University of Michigan indicates that cigarette smoking depresses the reflexes. A study of 45 healthy male students showed that reflex response was reduced sharply within a minute after smoking was started and that the reduction was as much as 67 percent within four minutes after the subject started smoking a high-nicotine cigarette. A similar but less pronounced effect was noted when low-nicotine cigarettes were smoked. No reflex depression occurred when nicotine-free lettuce cigarettes were smoked. Reflexes began to return to normal soon after smoking was stopped, but it usually took a full 20 minutes before the presmoking level was regained. When a subject started smoking a second cigarette, a similar pattern appeared.[6]

[5] Harold A. Solomon, Roger Priore, and Irving Bross, ''Cigarette Smoking and Periodontal Disease,'' Journal of the American Dental Association, vol. 77, p. 1081, November, 1968.

[6] Edward F. Domino and Alana M. Von Baumgarten, ''Effects of Smoking Cigarettes of Differing Nicotine Content on the Human Patellar Reflex.''
Paper presented at the 52nd Meeting of the Federation of American Societies for Experimental Biology in Atlantic City, N.J., Apr. 16, 1968.

A different type of study, which provides another possible explanation for the high rate of traffic accidents of cigarette smokers, was reported at the 1968 meeting of the American Chemical Society by investigators from the U.S. Public Health Service's National Air Control Administration laboratories in Cincinnati. These studies show that carbon monoxide which has been inhaled with cigarette smoke may not be completely eliminated from the blood even more than six hours after a person stops smoking. In fact, in some smokers the level of carbon monoxide in the blood drops only about 30 percent overnight. When carbon monoxide inhalation from heavy traffic is added to this, a dangerously high level of carbon monoxide in the blood may result.

The slowing of reflex response and the increase of carbon monoxide in the blood, as well as the distracting aspects of cigarette smoking, could all contribute to the higher accident rates of drivers who smoke.

TOBACCO --- ILLNESS & DISABILITY

Physicians have long suspected that the use of tobacco—particularly cigarette smoking—contributes to illness and disability, but only in recent years have studies confirmed this impression and measured its importance and its magnitude.

In the previous chapter we noted the colossal and increasing amount of disability caused by emphysema—14,000 new victims disabled each year and a predicted 20 million workers disabled by 1975—most of this attributable to cigarette smoking.

Thirty years ago the Life Extension Institute of New York reported that the examination records of presumably healthy persons showed that smokers complained of cough 300 percent more often than nonsmokers; of nose and throat trouble, 167 percent more often; of palpitations, 50 percent more often; of pain over the heart, 73 percent more often; of heartburn, 100 percent more often; and of nervousness, 76 percent more often.[1]

The American Cancer Society's prospective studies indicate that men aged 40 to 69 who are heavy cigarette smokers are hospitalized 50 percent more frequently than nonsmokers.

Studies by the California State Department of Public Health reveal that activity limitation and days of disability occasioned by chronic conditions are substantially greater among men aged 25 through 64 who smoke cigarettes than among nonsmokers. Similarly, the frequency of such conditions as cough was much higher among cigarette smokers.

In England a study of school children 11 to 18 years of age revealed that even at this early age boys and girls who smoke cigarettes have more respiratory illnesses with persistent cough, phlegm, etc., than those who do not smoke; that the more a child smokes, the more likely he is to have such symptoms; and that these symptoms decrease promptly with cessation of smoking.

A COMPREHENSIVE STUDY

Although limited studies like those summarized above indicate a significant relationship of cigarette smoking to illness and disability as well as to early death, the first major comprehensive survey of this relationship was reported by the Surgeon General of the U.S. Public Health Service in 1967. This survey was started in July, 1964, as a new portion of the National Health Survey inaugurated in 1957 and has been carried on continuously since that time.

In carrying out this survey, interviewers each year visit 42,000 families in various parts of the country, scientifically selected as

[1] "The Effects of Tobacco Smoking," Proceedings of the Life Extension Institute, p. 55, May–June, 1939.

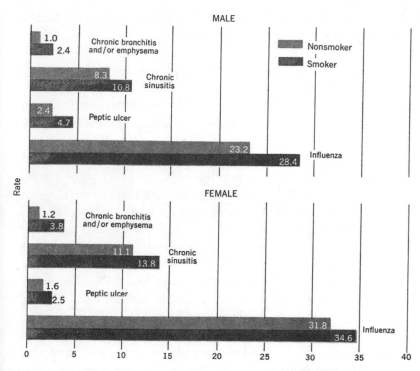

Figure 9.1. *Illness from bronchitis, emphysema, sinusitis, peptic ulcer, and influenza: smokers versus nonsmokers, males and females, fiscal year 1965. (Rates per 100 persons per year.) (Source: U.S. Public Health Service Publication No. 1,000, May 1967.)*

representative in proper proportions of all elements of the noninstitutionalized population of the United States. The purpose of this National Health Survey is to collect health and related information about the American people to aid in the assessment of health problems and in the formulation of health programs.

In this survey all families were questioned about illnesses, disability, and days absent from work because of illness, as well as the nature of the illness. During the year beginning July 1, 1964, interviewers inquired—after all other questions about health had been answered—about the smoking habits of persons in the family who were seventeen years of age or over.

Three major conclusions emerged from this study:

1 Members of the nation's labor force who smoke cigarettes spend over a third again as much time away from their jobs because of illness as persons who have never smoked cigarettes.

2 Women who smoke cigarettes, including both housewives and those who work outside the home, spend 17 percent more days ill in bed than women who have never smoked.

3 For the nation as a whole, there are now 77 million "excess" lost workdays associated with cigarette smoking each year. ("Excess" days are days lost which would not have been lost if cigarette smokers had the same rates as people who have never smoked cigarettes.) The excess loss of 77 million workdays represents almost 20 percent of the entire annual work loss from illness in the United States.

Some other highlights and interpretations of the results of this study are given below.

Chronic conditions

Chronic conditions are those illnesses which last for a long time— months, even years. Asthma, tuberculosis, rheumatic fever, heart disease, cancer, chronic bronchitis, emphysema, diabetes and arthritis are all chronic illnesses. In the Health Interview Survey, any other illness which began more than 3 months before the time of the interview was also considered a chronic illness.

In the 1964–1965 survey both male and female cigarette smokers reported more cases of chronic illness than those who never smoked. There was a higher rate of chronic illness among the heavy smokers than among those who smoked fewer cigarettes or

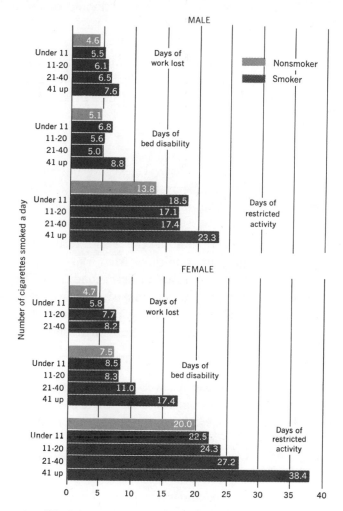

Figure 9.2. *Work loss days, restricted activity days, and bed disability days attributable to sickness: smokers versus nonsmokers, males and females, fiscal year 1965. (Rates by number of cigarettes per day.) (Source: U.S. Public Health Service Publication No. 1,000, May 1967.)*

none at all. Smokers also reported more chronic conditions per person than persons who never smoked.

There are 11 million more cases of chronic illness yearly in this country than would exist if all individuals had the same rate of sickness as those who had never smoked cigarettes.

Heart disease

According to the Surgeon General's Report on Smoking and Health, "Male cigarette smokers have a higher death rate from coronary artery disease than non-smoking males. . . ."

The health survey data confirm the same relationship with regard to illness from heart conditions. Men who have smoked at some time in their lives had a rate of heart conditions 22 percent higher than those who had never smoked; men who over some period of time smoked more than two packs of cigarettes a day reported 93 percent more heart conditions than those who never smoked.

There are 280,000 more persons who report having heart trouble in this country than there would be if all people had the same rate as those who never smoked.

Chronic bronchitis and emphysema

The 1964 Report to the Surgeon General found a relationship between smoking and chronic bronchitis and emphysema. The Health Interview Survey shows the extent of this relationship as far as illness is concerned. Male smokers have a rate of illness from these diseases more than double the rate for males who have never smoked, and women smokers three times the rate for women who have never smoked.

In all, there are over 1 million more cases of chronic bronchitis and/or emphysema in the nation than there would be if all people had the same rate as those who never smoked.

Sinusitis

The nasal condition of stuffiness and mucopurulent discharge, commonly called *sinusitis*, may seem to the nonafflicted to be a minor illness. However, to the person suffering from it, this condition—an inflammation of the lining of the nasal sinuses—can be very distressing and disabling. There has long been clinical evidence that smoking aggravates this condition and that meaningful relief can be obtained when the patient stops smoking.

The Health Interview Survey revealed that heavy smokers report sinusitis 75 percent more frequently than people who have never smoked.

There are 1.8 million more cases of sinusitis in this country every year than there would be if all people had the same rate as those who never smoked.

Peptic ulcer

Epidemiological studies indicate a close association between cigarette smoking and peptic ulcers. Of these the incidence of ulcers of the stomach is greater than the incidence of ulcers of the duodenum.

The number of cases of peptic ulcers reported in the 1964–1965 Health Interview Survey was almost 100 percent higher for male smokers and more than 50 percent higher for female smokers than for male and female nonsmokers, respectively. The difference in rates was more marked as the number of cigarettes smoked increased.

There are 1 million more cases of peptic ulcers each year in this country than there would be if all people had the same rate as those who never smoked.

Lung cancer

Illness from lung cancer was not reported in the study because there are comparatively few people ill with this disease at any one time. In a study in Connecticut (1935–1951) it was found that the percent of men surviving 3, 6, and 12 months after a diagnosis was approximately 45 percent, 26 percent, and 13 percent, respectively. "Five-year cures" were almost nonexistent.

Smoking patterns

About 51 percent of the men and 33 percent of the women included in the National Health Survey were found to be cigarette smokers and another 19 percent of the men and 8 percent of the women were former cigarette smokers. The former smokers, for the most part, reported poorer health than smokers. The obvious reason for this is that the group of ex-smokers contains many ill persons who gave up smoking because of illness.

In addition to recording smoking characteristics by "present smokers," "former smokers," and "never smoked," the survey also recorded numbers of cigarettes smoked per day—both the "heaviest amount" smoked during the person's lifetime and the "present amount" smoked at the time of the survey. Full breakdowns of these classifications and their relationship to illness may be found in the report.[2]

---

[2] "Cigarette Smoking and Health Characteristics—United States—July 1964 to June 1965," U.S. Department of Health, Education, and Welfare, Washington, May, 1967; and "Smoking and Illness," a pamphlet summarizing the above report, National Clearinghouse for Smoking and Health, U.S. Public Health Service, Washington, 1968.

Days lost

The National Health Survey is concerned with three measures of the impact of illness. (See Table 9.1.)

Days lost from work These are days absent from job or business because of illness or injury. They involve only those who are currently employed. In the survey year, there were 399 million workdays lost in the United States because of illness. A total of 77 million days, or 19 percent, were excess workdays lost because of the higher rates which exist among persons who have ever smoked cigarettes regularly as compared with those who never smoked.

Bed days These are days when the person is sufficiently ill or disabled as to spend all or most of the day in bed, either at home or in a hospital. For the entire population 17 years of age and older there were 853 million bed days in the survey year. A total of 88 million of these days, or 10 percent, were "excess" days, lost because of the higher rates which exist among persons who have

TABLE 9.1 **Illness and disability by amount of smoking (percent increase over nonsmokers)**

		Cigarettes smoked per day		
		½ to 1 pack	1 to 2 packs	2+ packs
Days lost from work	Men	+30%	+48%	+83%
	Women	+60	+79	+140
Bed days	Men	+22	+22	+53
	Women	+17	+57	+192
Restricted activity	Men	+32	+39	+81
	Women	+22	+48	+146

SOURCE: See footnote 2, page 106.

ever smoked cigarettes regularly as compared with those who never smoked.

Days of restricted activity These are days when a person cuts down his usual activities for as much as a day because of an illness or an injury. There were 2,369 million such days in the survey year; 306 million, or 13 percent, were excess days lost because of the higher rates which exist among persons who have ever smoked cigarettes regularly as compared with those who never smoked.

The costs The cost of medical care and hospitalization for these excess illnesses and the economic loss from the disability attributable to cigarette smoking are impossible to compute accurately, but the total would certainly be staggering. It is reported that some corporations and businesses are beginning to discourage smoking because of the loss of time and the risk of disability and early death of valuable personnel.[3] The findings presented in this chapter suggest that cigarette smokers should be charged higher rates than nonsmokers for disability insurance and hospital insurance as well as for life insurance.

EFFECTS UPON NONSMOKERS
OF BREATHING TOBACCO SMOKE

The editorial in *Science* quoted on page 52 states: "When an individual smokes in a poorly ventilated space in the presence of others, he infringes the rights of others and becomes a serious contributor to air pollution." What effect the inhalation of such smoke-polluted air has upon others is a question frequently asked, but upon which it is difficult to obtain definitive information.

Physicians have long known that some individuals are made uncomfortable or acutely ill by exposure to tobacco smoke. A clinical

---

3 "Top Executives Heed Warning to Stop Smoking," Minneapolis Tribune, May 14, 1967.

study of this phenomenon, made by the Pediatric Allergy Service of the University of Kansas Medical Center, concludes that intolerance to tobacco smoke is common in both allergic and non-allergic patients, and that the most common complaints are eye irritation, nasal symptoms (sneezing, blocking, discharge, itching, and dryness), headache, and cough. It also concludes that the effects of tobacco smoke appear to be of an irritative rather than an allergic character: "The many individuals who develop symptoms from tobacco smoke need the understanding and support of the physician in helping them to avoid its noxious effects." [4]

A different type of study, dealing with the effects of exposure of children to tobacco smoke, has been released by a team of investigators at Wayne State University in Detroit. This study compares the number of acute illnesses among children under 16 years of age in homes in which there is parental smoking, with the number of illnesses of children in homes in which parents do not smoke. The results show that rates of acute illnesses (mostly respiratory) among smokers' children are approximately twice as high as among nonsmokers' children. There is also some evidence that the amount of smoke in the home environment may be related to the chance of illness. This study confirms the results of a similar study, made in Denver and reported in 1967 by the senior investigator.[5] The subject is of great importance and it is hoped, as the investigators state, that these studies will be extended and repeated.

[4] Frederick Speer, "Tobacco and the Non-Smoker," Archives of Environmental Health, vol. 16, p. 443, March, 1968.
[5] Paul Cameron et al., "The Health of Smokers' and Non-Smokers' Children—Preliminary Report I." Press release and personal communication, October, 1968.

DISSENTING OPINIONS

The tobacco industry and a few independent physicians take issue with the accepted conclusions about the health damage caused by cigarette smoking and keep making statements or raising questions such as the following:

Since the cause of cancer is not known, how can it be said that cigarette smoking causes lung cancer?

While it is true that the basic cause or causes of cancer are not known, it does not follow that contributory causes are not important. No one disputes the fact that x-rays and atomic radiation and even excessive exposure to sunlight cause cancer. Neither is there any dispute about the relationship of high blood pressure to strokes or the relationship of overweight to diabetes even though the cause of high blood pressure and the cause of diabetes are unknown. Likewise, we frequently refer to the means by which a disease is acquired as its cause: for example, although the cause of rabies (hydrophobia) is a virus, most people say that rabies is caused by the bite of a rabid (mad) animal, usually a dog. Furthermore, many measures for the prevention of disease were accepted and employed long before the cause of the disease was known. In 1848, when Dr. John Snow observed that most of the victims of a cholera epidemic in London had used water from the Broad Street pump, he identified the source of the disease even though the cause of cholera had not yet been discovered; then when he removed the handle of this pump, the epidemic subsided. When Dr. William Jenner of England noted in the latter part of the eighteenth century that milkmaids rarely contracted smallpox, while almost everyone else did, he suspected that a mild disease called cowpox frequently contracted from cattle might be protecting them. Experiments proved this to be true, and he started to vaccinate people against smallpox in 1796. The virus that causes smallpox, however, was not identified until 1892.

The observation of a British ship's doctor during long voyages led in 1795 to the issue of fresh fruit and fruit juices to prevent scurvy among the crews. We now know that scurvy is due to a deficiency of vitamin C, but this fact was not discovered until more than a century later. Likewise, water purification was used to prevent typhoid fever, and screening against mosquitos to prevent malaria and yellow fever, long before the *causes* of these diseases were known.

There is no substance in tobacco smoke that has been proved to cause cancer, heart disease, or emphysema.

This is literally true, but it is not true that cigarette smoke, which is a mixture of many toxic chemicals, does not cause these diseases. Statements such as these are half true and half untrue. In this sense they are, like half bricks, more destructive than whole bricks because they carry farther.

The evidence is only statistical and therefore inconclusive.

Statistics, according to Webster's *New World Dictionary*, are numerical facts assembled and classified so as to present significant information. The above argument, therefore, is meaningless to anyone familiar with the scientific method. In fact, most conclusions in scientific work are based upon the analysis of data, that is, upon statistics. It is by the use of statistics that the Department of Agriculture is able to report the average number of cigarettes sold per person per year. Tobacco companies spend more than $300 million a year to advertise cigarettes. Being efficient business organizations, these companies must have evidence—statistical evidence—that this enormous expenditure pays off. In medical and biological studies cause-and-effect relationships are judged on the basis of extent and consistency of association and relevant information supporting the interpretation of such relationships. Concerning this, Dr. Warren Weaver, president of the Alfred P. Sloan Foundation and former director for medical sciences of the Rockefeller Foundation, wrote: "The automatic discarding of evidence because it is statistical is unscientific and wholly unwarranted. Statistical evidence is, in essentially all non-trivial cases, the only sort of evidence we can possibly have."

Examples of conclusions based upon human statistical observations are the relation of the drug thalidomide taken by women during pregnancy to the development of deformed babies; the relation of a deficiency of iodine in one's food and drink to the development of goiter; the relation of exposure to radiation, whether from x-rays or from atomic fallout, to cancer; the relation of obesity to diabetes and heart disease. It is by the use of statistics that we know that vaccination protects against poliomyelitis, smallpox, measles, etc., that drugs are of value for the prevention or treatment of various diseases, that surgery and x-ray treatments save the lives of many cancer patients, and that certain drugs help or even cure some cancer patients.

There may be a genetic factor which causes a person to smoke and also causes him to develop lung cancer, coronary heart disease, or emphysema.

This is an hypothesis without supportive evidence and one that is inconsistent with established facts. For example, such an hypothesis cannot account for the increases in these diseases in recent years, for the parallelism between their increase and the increase in cigarette smoking, for the much higher death rates among cigarette smokers than among cigar or pipe smokers, or for the reduction in deaths among former cigarette smokers who have discontinued the habit.

The statistical evidence is not supported by animal experimentation.

As Lord Robert Platt, President of the Royal College of Physicians of London, has pointed out, the conclusion that cigarette smoking causes lung cancer, chronic bronchitis, and heart disease is based upon extensive animal experimentation, with the best possible animal for such an experiment: namely, *man*. Those who make this statement doubtless refer to experiments on laboratory animals. It is true that until recently lung cancer had not been produced in laboratory animals by exposing them to cigarette smoke. However, a report from the Imperial Cancer Research Fund of London in December, 1967, states that some mice that breathed a cigarette smoke-air mixture for 12 minutes every other day developed lung cancer. Dogs that have been taught to inhale cigarette smoke through a tube develop bronchitis and emphysema, and their lungs contain abnormal cells of the type considered precancerous in humans. The probability is that if they do not die earlier from other diseases, these dogs eventually will develop lung cancer.

However, even if animals that have been taught to smoke should not develop lung cancer or the other diseases associated with smoking, it would not disprove the conclusion that cigarette smoking causes these diseases in man. It is well known that animals react differently to infectious agents, to toxins, and to drugs. For example, carbon tetrachloride produces many tumors in mice but none in rats; dimethylaminoazobenzene ("butter yellow") produces cancer of the liver in rats but not in hamsters; the "polyoma virus" causes a wide variety of tumors in different animals; compounds of beryllium cause pulmonary cancer in certain animals but not in others; and laboratory animals are not susceptible to various diseases of man such as smallpox, typhoid fever, and measles.

It is unreasonable to believe that cigarette smoking could cause lung cancer, cancer of the bladder, coronary thrombosis, chronic bronchitis, emphysema, etc.

To the uninformed this point may seem well taken, but few diseases or poisons affect only one organ or system in the body. Typhoid fever and syphilis affect practically all body organs and systems; diphtheria toxin acts on the central nervous system to produce paralysis and also causes serious damage to heart muscles; and nearly all chemical poisons have multiple effects on the body —phenol poisoning causes disturbances of the digestive tract, nervous disorders, mental aberrations and eruptions of the skin, with death resulting from damage to the liver and kidneys; and bichloride of mercury produces ulcers of the mouth, loss of teeth, necrosis of the jaw, skin eruptions, loss of weight, affliction of the nervous system with tremors, weakness, hallucinations and mental deterioration. Furthermore, cigarette smoke contains several different chemical agents, each with its own possible ill effects.

Not all cigarette smokers or even heavy smokers develop lung cancer or the other diseases that are associated with smoking.

To a physician this is not at all surprising, because individual differences in susceptibility and resistance to disease are much more common than uniform reactions. For example, less than 2 percent of persons infected with the poliomyelitis virus develop paralysis. Yet no one doubts that poliomyelitis is caused by a virus. Likewise, not everyone exposed to the tubercle bacillus gets tuberculosis; nor does everyone exposed to measles, venereal diseases, influenza, or even smallpox contract these diseases.

Furthermore, even the fact that many long-time smokers show no obvious ill effects does not disprove the harmfulness of smoking. The lucky few are the exceptions to the rule. Most persons with syphilis become incapacitated and eventually die from the effects of the disease upon the cardiovascular system, the brain, or some other vital organ. However, some syphilitics live to advanced age and die from other causes. No one would suggest that because of this, syphilis is not a serious and frequently a fatal disease.

Since there is increasing evidence that viruses may cause human cancer, how could cigarette smoking be a cause?

The answer is that even if a virus should prove to be involved in the development of lung cancer, cigarette smoking could be a trigger mechanism that upsets a balance between the virus and the body cells, thus leading to the development of cancer. This is apparently what occurs with *herpes labialis* or "cold sores"—a disease caused by a virus that is continuously present in the body but causes trouble only when the balance between the virus and the cells of the skin is upset by local irritation, such as a common cold or sunburn or windburn.

Cigarette smoking cannot be a cause of coronary heart disease, bronchitis, emphysema, and lung cancer because other causes have been demonstrated.

While a number of other known and probably some unknown factors contribute to the development of coronary heart disease, emphysema, and even lung cancer, this in no way negates or detracts from the importance of cigarette smoking as a causative factor in these diseases.

Life expectancy has been increasing in spite of increased cigarette smoking.

In the past decade the life expectancy in this country has increased less than half a year. And it is not likely to increase until cigarette smoking is reduced. (See Table 4.2.) Furthermore, the average life expectancy of men aged 25 who smoke less than a pack a day is 5 years less and of men who smoke two or more packs a day 8 years less than the life expectancy of nonsmokers of the same age.

Cancer of the lung is more frequent than cancer of the mouth or the larynx, which are more heavily exposed to cigarette smoke than is the lung. Also cancer of the lung occurs most frequently in certain areas of the lung while cigarette smoke reaches all portions of the lung.

It is well known that the tissues of the body show varying degrees of susceptibility to infection and to irritant substances. This certainly is true also of the tissues of the mouth, the larynx, and the lung in regard to their exposure to cigarette smoke. The fact that lung cancer develops most frequently in certain areas of the lung is not surprising; the same phenomenon occurs in pneumonia, tuberculosis, and other diseases. This fact is in no way related to the cause of the disease.

Lung cancer is much more frequent in men than in women, yet women smoke almost as much as men.

The explanation for this is either that there is a sex difference in susceptibility to lung cancer as is true for cancer of the breast, cancer of the stomach, and certain other types of cancer, or that women have not smoked as long as men and in the past have not smoked as much or inhaled as regularly.

The reported increases in deaths from lung cancer and emphysema are due to better diagnosis and do not represent an actual increase in these diseases.

This argument has been disproved many times by studies based on diagnoses made at autopsy. Certainly there has been no change in the ability of pathologists to diagnose lung cancer at autopsy.

At the congressional hearings on the cigarette-labeling bill, 39 of the 49 medical authorities and statisticians who testified disagreed with the report of the Surgeon General's Advisory Committee and charged that its findings were distorted.

This statement ignores the fact that the 10 physicians who agreed with the conclusions of the Surgeon General's report and testified in support of cigarette-labeling legislation were representatives of national medical and health organizations with tens of thousands of physician members, while the 39 who testified as indicated above were sought out and presumably compensated as consultants by the tobacco industry. Concerning this testimony the Chairman of the Senate Commerce Committee which conducted these hearings said: [1]

> There remains no reasonable doubt that cigarette smoking is a significant health hazard. Fifteen years have passed since the first substantial research clearly identified smoking as the cause of lung cancer and other diseases. During that 15 years, despite the frenzied efforts of the industry to exonerate the cigarette, new evidence has confirmed the verdict.
>
> The Commerce Committee held 10 days of hearings on smoking and health. While we heard from a number of individual physicians who remain unconvinced by the evidence, we found that no disinterested medical or scientific body which has investigated the relationship between smoking and dis-

---

[1] From Congressional Record, U.S. Senate, p. 13405, June 16, 1965.

ease, has failed to conclude that cigarette smoking is a serious health hazard.

Above all, we were faced with the unanimous verdict of the Advisory Committee to the Surgeon General of the U.S. Public Health Service—the Committee of 10 physicians and scientists whose competence and whose freedom from bias has never been questioned. On January 11, 1964, after nearly 2 years of study, this select committee concluded: Cigarette smoking is a health hazard of sufficient importance in the United States to warrant appropriate remedial action.

The subjects of the American Cancer Society studies do not represent a true cross section of the population. Therefore, one is not justified in drawing conclusions from these studies.

The first part of this statement is true; the second part is false. The subjects of these studies were friends or acquaintances of 68,000 American Cancer Society volunteers in 1,121 counties of 25 states. The group therefore consisted primarily of what are usually described as "average Americans." There were some, but relatively few, from the migrant, institutionalized, uneducated, and lowest socioeconomic strata of our society. This, however, does not detract from the validity of the conclusions since both smokers and nonsmokers were from the same population group. In fact, if a similar study had been made of individuals in the lowest stratum, the death rates would have been even higher because there is more smoking and more illness in this group.

There has been no scientific proof that cigarette smoking causes any human disease.

The answer to this statement is contained in the various studies reported in this book. The diseases attributable to smoking are more frequent in smokers than in nonsmokers. They increase with dosage, that is, with the number of cigarettes smoked daily, with the degree of inhalation, and with the age at which smoking was begun; *and* the risk of developing these diseases decreases with the discontinuance of smoking. The tars in cigarette smoke produce skin cancer in animals; the nicotine affects the cardiovascular system; and cigarette smoke has produced lung cancer in mice and produces emphysema in dogs. Furthermore, there is no explanation other than one of cause and effect for the consistent association of these diseases with cigarette smoking.

WHO SMOKES & WHY?

CHAPTER ELEVEN

Until thirty or forty years ago smoking was limited almost exclusively to men. Boys and occasionally girls experimented with cigarettes but few smoked regularly. The few women who smoked did so mostly in the privacy of their homes.

SMOKING IN THE GENERAL POPULATION

Today the situation is vastly different. According to the National Health Survey of 1964–1965, 51 percent of the men and 33 percent of women over 17 years of age are cigarette smokers. An estimated 19 percent of men have discontinued smoking and 30 percent never smoked cigarettes regularly. Of the women 8 percent were former smokers and 59 percent had never smoked regularly. In older age groups the percentage of smokers was substantially lower in both sexes than in younger groups. This is due in part to a discontinuance of smoking and in part to the fact that when these individuals were young, smoking was not so prevalent as it is today. As a result, fewer boys and girls became habituated smokers. The relation of smoking habits by sex to age, residence, color, family income, and education, as indicated by the National Health Survey, is shown in Table 11.1

TABLE 11.1 Cigarette smoking by sex, age, residence,

Characteristic	MALES		
	Never smoked regularly	Former smokers	Present smokers
Total	29.9%	19.2%	50.7%
Age			
17–24	44.1	6.6	48.6
25–34	24.6	14.7	60.7
35–44	21.2	20.5	58.1
45–54	22.2	21.9	55.8
55–64	26.3	27.0	46.5
65 up	43.4	28.0	28.4
Residence			
Metropolitan †	29.8	19.3	50.7
City ‡	28.4	19.5	52.0
Farm §	37.3	17.9	44.8
Color			
White	29.7	20.1	50.0
Nonwhite	31.1	11.6	57.1
Family Income			
Under $3,000	27.1	18.1	54.9
3,000–4,999	27.6	17.5	54.8
5,000–6,999	29.0	18.7	52.2
7,000–9,999	30.1	20.4	49.3
10,000 up	34.1	22.0	43.9
Education			
Under 5 years	27.4	19.3	53.2
5–8 years	24.3	20.1	55.5
9–12 years	30.1	17.6	52.2
13 years and up	36.3	22.6	41.1

SMOKING BY YOUNG PEOPLE

A questionnaire survey of 6,459 students in 16 high schools published in the April, 1967, issue of *Scholastic Roto*—a national
magazine supplement for high school newspapers—reported that

color, family income, and education *

FEMALES

Never smoked regularly	Former smokers	Present smokers
58.3%	7.9%	33.5%
59.7	5.5	33.9
46.4	9.8	43.5
46.6	9.5	43.6
53.0	9.3	37.4
67.2	7.6	24.9
85.2	4.5	9.5
55.0	8.3	36.4
62.0	7.5	30.1
78.4	4.6	16.4
57.9	8.1	33.7
62.3	5.9	31.2
63.2	5.3	31.1
59.8	7.2	32.8
57.8	8.6	33.3
55.4	9.4	34.9
53.1	10.3	36.3
72.3	3.0	24.4
64.8	4.8	30.0
55.9	8.4	35.5
53.7	12.0	34.1

* Age-adjusted percent distributions for number of present cigarette smokers, former smokers, and nonsmokers, male and female, 17 years of age and older, 1965 fiscal year.

† "Metropolitan area" refers to the Census Standard Metropolitan Statistical Area (SMSA) classification.

‡ City refers to the Census classification: outside SMSA, nonfarm.

§ Farm refers to the Census classification: outside SMSA, farm.

SOURCE: Unpublished data from Health Interview Survey, National Center for Health Statistics, Public Health Service, U.S. Department of Health, Education, and Welfare.

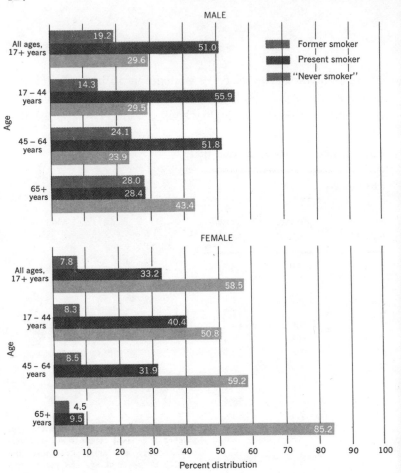

Figure 11.1. *Percent distribution of the population 17 years of age and over, by smoking status according to sex and age. (Source: "Cigarette Smoking and Health Characteristics—July 1964 to June 1965," U.S. Public Health Service, May 1967.)*

94 percent of the students said that they believe smoking is harmful. In spite of this, 44 percent of high school boys and 37 percent of high school girls smoke. As sophomores 38 percent of boys and 27 percent of girls smoke. By the senior year the percentage of smokers increases to 46 percent for boys and 42 percent for girls.

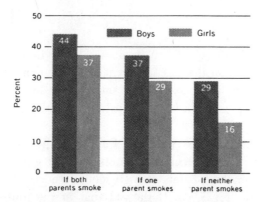

Figure 11.2. *Teen-age smoking linked to parental smoking.* (*Source:* Cancer Facts and Figures, *American Cancer Society, 1965.*)

In 1957 an intensive study of smoking among high school students was made for the American Cancer Society by Dr. Daniel Horn. The study involved 11,060 boys and 10,920 girls. The percentage of boys and girls who smoked is shown, by grade, in Table 11.2. The general results of this study, as summarized in the *American Journal of Public Health,* were:

1 The percentage of smokers was highest among children of families in which both parents smoked cigarettes, lowest in families in which neither parent smoked, and intermediate in families in which only one parent smoked.

2 The smoking behavior of boys tended to conform more closely to that of the father, while the smoking pattern of girls followed more closely that of the mother.

3 The percentage of smokers among children from families in which one or both parents continued to smoke was significantly higher than the percentage in which one or both parents had given up smoking.

4 Each successive school grade had a higher percentage of smokers.

5 The percentage of smokers was higher among students in Catholic schools than among students in the city public

schools. It was lowest among students in the suburban schools.

6 The percentage of smokers among boys who did not participate in athletics was substantially higher than among those who did. The percentage of smokers was higher also among students who did not participate in any school activities.[1]

At the meeting of the American Public Health Association in October, 1967, a University of Illinois research group reported a study of the smoking habits of high school students in Rockford, Illinois, a city of 125,000. It showed that in the ninth grade 19 percent of students smoked; in the tenth grade 22 percent; in the eleventh grade 26 percent; and in the twelfth grade 30 percent; also that a higher percentage of boys smoked than of girls in all grades. A comparison with earlier studies suggests that an increasing proportion of students are beginning to smoke at younger ages and that the percentage of high school girls who smoke is progressively approaching that of boys.[2]

TABLE 11.2 Smoking by high school students (percentage of regular smokers by grade)

	Boys	Girls
Freshmen	14.5%	4.6%
Sophomores	25.2	10.6
Juniors	31.1	16.2
Seniors	35.4	26.2

SOURCE: See footnote 1.

[1] Daniel Horn, F. A. Courts, R. M. Taylor, and E. S. Saloman, "Cigarette Smoking among High School Students," American Journal of Public Health, vol. 49, p. 1497, November, 1959.
[2] W. N. Creswell et al., "A 1967 Replica of the Horn Study of Smoking Youth," presented at the American Public Health Association Meeting in Miami Beach, Fla., Oct. 26, 1967. Abstract: "Smoking and Health," Public Health Reports, vol. 83, p. 224, March, 1968.

A nationwide survey of smoking by boys and girls each year of age from 12 to 18 was reported in 1968 by the National Clearing-house for Smoking and Health. Among the findings of this survey were that: [3]

1 The proportion of teen-agers who smoke appears to have declined appreciably from the levels reported in numerous studies over the past ten years. For the percentage of smokers by age and sex, see Table 11.3.

2 Of the teen-agers 45 percent said that they definitely do not expect to be smokers in five years; another 34 percent said that they probably will not be smokers then; 6 percent said that they have no opinion about this; only 12 percent said they probably will be smokers within five years. Even if those who said that they do not know what to expect are included with those who expect to be smokers, the expectation is that only 23 percent of the boys and 18 percent of the girls will be smokers when this group is aged 17 to 23. This is about half the proportion of smokers reported in recent years for these age groups.

TABLE 11.3 Proportion of teen-agers who are regular smokers, by age and sex

Age	Boys			Girls		
	Weekly	Daily	Combined	Weekly	Daily	Combined
12	1.0%	0.3%	1.3%	0.3%	0%	0.3%
13	0.6	1.0	1.6	0	0.6	0.6
14	1.2	4.4	5.6	0.3	0.6	0.9
15	2.9	10.7	13.6	1.8	5.6	7.4
16	2.9	17.4	20.3	3.6	8.3	11.9
17	6.0	19.6	25.6	3.9	11.8	15.7
18	4.1	31.4	35.5	3.9	17.4	21.3
	2.7%	12.0%	14.7%	2.0%	6.4%	8.4%

SOURCE: See footnote 3.

[3] Daniel Horn, "Current Smoking among Teenagers," Public Health Reports, vol. 83, No. 6, p. 458, June, 1968.

3   There is an overwhelming awareness among youth at each year of age from 12 to 18 that cigarette smoking is a health hazard.

4   Smoking is more common among children in families in which there is smoking.

5   There is more smoking among the "out group" in the school setting, that is, those who have slipped behind their age-mates in school and do not expect to go on to college, than among the rest of the school population.

6   There is less smoking among parents of high school students than was reported in previous studies. This suggests that smoking by parents and by their teen-age children influence each other.

Other surveys of smokers and nonsmokers in high schools and colleges indicate that, although there are many exceptions, cigarette smokers as a group participate less than nonsmokers in athletics and other extracurricular activities, have lower IQs, are inferior students, are predominantly from lower social and economic backgrounds, and come from homes in which one or both parents smoke.

SMOKING AMONG COLLEGE STUDENTS

A report from the University of Washington in Seattle showed that in the class which entered in 1964 only 13 percent of the boys and 10 percent of the girls smoked.

A 1965 survey of freshmen students who entered the University of Illinois in the fall of 1964 indicated that 40 percent smoked cigarettes. Of these, 43 percent said that they would like to stop. Grades showed an inverse relationship to smoking: of students with an A average, only 17 percent smoked, while 59 percent of students with an E average smoked.

At Princeton University, which has long kept a record of smoking by entering freshmen, there has been a persistent downward trend in the percentage of cigarette smokers, with the surprisingly low figure of 7 percent in 1966. (See Table 11.4.)

An analysis of the level of education in relation to smoking habits was made by Hammond and Garfinkel in their study of a million men and women. It revealed that in males the smallest percentage of smokers is among college graduates; the highest among high school dropouts. The rates among college dropouts are slightly higher than among high school graduates. In females, the college graduates and the group with no high school education tended to have a smaller percentage of cigarette smokers than other groups. The differences, however, are not great.

Other conclusions of this study are that a larger proportion of college graduates than of the less educated have *given up* smoking and that a larger proportion of college graduates smoke low-tar, low-nicotine cigarettes. The proportion of cigarette smoking is lower among farmers, teachers, lawyers, clergymen, doctors, dentists, and veterinarians than in the general population. The proportion of ex-smokers and of men smoking low-tar, low-

TABLE 11.4 **Cigarette smoking by Princeton University freshmen, 1948–1966**

Year	Percentage
1948	42
1952	30
1962	23
1963	15
1965	10
1966	7

nicotine cigarettes is higher in these occupational groups (except farmers) than in the general population.[4]

Other studies show that the greatest amount of smoking is by men in lower socioeconomic groups. In other words, those who smoke most are the ones who can least afford either the cost of cigarettes, for which the average smoker spends $150 to $300 a year, or—and this is vastly more important—the cost of the illnesses and the disabilities that result from smoking. Dr. Philippe Shubik, a committee chairman of the International Union Against Cancer, noting the decrease in smoking among the better educated, said: "It seems that the more intelligent people have decided to preserve themselves and the more stupid to eliminate themselves."

In a special article entitled "Top Executives Heed Warnings to Stop Smoking," James Schwartz, of the *Minneapolis Tribune*, wrote that at some Twin City corporations heavy smokers are beginning to heed the warnings of health groups. "There is definitely a trend away from smoking here," said a Honeywell, Inc., executive: "The younger men—the sharper types—seem to be especially influenced by recent smoking reports." His remarks were confirmed by a Pillsbury Company source who said cigarette smoking there is becoming a "woman's vice," partly because of company concern for employee health. Top decision makers—and younger men who aspire to the role—represent important investments.

This article goes on to quote Dr. Frank Martin, a private physician: "It's unusual to find a top executive who smokes cigarettes these days.—I'm impressed also by the great numbers of ambitious young men who have shunned the habit." [5]

[4] E. C. Hammond and Lawrence Garfinkel, "Smoking Habits of Men and Women," Journal of the National Cancer Institute, vol. 27, p. 435, August, 1961.
[5] James Schwartz, "Top Executives Heed Warnings to Stop Smoking," Minneapolis Tribune, May 14, 1967.

SMOKING BY PHYSICIANS

Of very special interest and significance are reports that relatively few physicians now smoke cigarettes. Fifteen years ago more than 60 percent of all physicians smoked cigarettes. Today it is about one-third of that percentage. In Massachusetts 52 percent of physicians were smoking in 1954; five years later only 38 percent were still smoking. In 1963, 33 percent of Rhode Island physicians were smoking cigarettes. On the basis of a nationwide questionnaire survey in early 1964 the journal *Modern Medicine* reported that of the 56,000 physicians who replied only 22.5 percent were then smoking cigarettes. Also in 1964 only 24 percent of Oregon physicians reported that they were smoking cigarettes.

Of 5,356 physicians in the American Cancer Society study of a million men and women, 66 percent gave a history of having been a regular cigarette smoker sometime in their lives. At the beginning of the study in 1959, 40 percent were smoking cigarettes. By 1965, this percentage had decreased to 29. A survey by the California Medical Association reported in January, 1968, indicates that 21 percent of the physicians in that state currently smoke cigarettes; 38 percent never smoked; and 1 percent did not report their smoking habits. Of physicians under 35 only 14 percent smoke cigarettes. Only 3 percent of California physicians said that they did not consider cigarette smoking a serious health hazard.

Even in Charlotte, N.C., according to a poll by the Charlotte *News* (March 16, 1968), only 15 percent of the physicians there still smoke cigarettes. Ninety-two percent said that they consider cigarette smoking harmful, 5 percent had no comment (or "didn't know" one way or the other), and only 3 percent did not think that smoking is harmful.

It is notable also that the greatest decreases in smoking by physicians have occurred among chest surgeons, pathologists, and radiologists—the physicians who specialize in the diagnosis and care of patients who suffer from diseases attributable to smoking.[6]

Nationwide it is estimated that 100,000 physicians have stopped smoking. Concerning this the U.S. Public Health Service says: "Maybe they know something you don't."

WHY PEOPLE SMOKE

The reasons people smoke are varied and complex. Learning to smoke is unpleasant for everyone and intolerable for many. It is only after one has developed a tolerance for tobacco that smoking ceases to be distressing, and it is not until one becomes habituated that smoking seems pleasurable.

For children who see their parents, teachers, other adults, and older brothers and sisters smoking, the desire to be like them, to be grown-up, constitutes a strong incentive to try it themselves. Studies show that children are much more likely to smoke if their parents smoke. An employee of a Minneapolis television station gave up smoking after seeing his four-year-old son test puff a discarded butt in the back yard. "That convinced me," he said. "All the statistics I've seen point to the fact that a child is likely to smoke if his parents do."

Many boys and girls start smoking to show their independence, as a symbol of revolt against authority, to feel sophisticated and grown-up, to be "one of the crowd," to gain social status, to have something to do. A junior high school paper of Queens, New York, put it this way: "Kids start smoking 'to be in'—the great urge of every teenager. Start smoking, after all it looks real hip and adult."

[6] "60,000 Answer MM Smoking Survey," Modern Medicine, Mar. 2, 1964, p. 18.

The advertisers of cigarettes exploit this urge by creating an image of a smoker as an outstanding athlete; a handsome, virile outdoor man; a nonchalant campus leader; a man who succeeds; a sophisticated, charming young woman.

For some smokers the motions and movements associated with smoking seem to have a soothing, pleasurable effect, similar to the chewing of tasteless objects such as pencils, straws, or chewing gum after the flavor is gone. It also seems that some of the satisfaction derived from smoking—particularly of pipes and cigars —is related to watching the smoke. Few people enjoy smoking in the dark, and blind men rarely smoke.

For persons who are self-conscious and insecure smoking provides an activity and something to do with their hands that takes their minds off themselves. Many accept the image created by cigarette advertisements of cigarette smoking as a symbol of poise, self-confidence, and social success. But once one becomes dependent upon cigarettes, habituation or addiction are impelling drives to continue.

Dr. Daniel Horn, Director of the National Clearinghouse for Smoking and Health, says that people smoke cigarettes for one or more of the following reasons: (1) for stimulation, such as to get started in the morning; (2) because of addiction; this smoker "must have" a cigarette after a certain amount of time has elapsed; (3) to reduce negative feelings, such as distress, anger, or fear; (4) out of habit—a behavior pattern followed almost involuntarily; (5) for oral gratification—the satisfaction derived from something in the mouth; and (6) for pleasurable relaxation —to enhance positive feelings, such as after a good dinner.

Dr. Horn feels that if a person analyzes his reasons for smoking, it may help him to break the habit.

Concerning the reasons for smoking and the associated behavioral problems, the World Conference on Smoking and Health concluded that much more knowledge is needed in this field and that investigators in the behavioral and social sciences, including communications and education, should be encouraged to conduct more extensive and intensive studies in this important area.

GIVING UP SMOKING [1]

CHAPTER TWELVE

The U.S. Public Health Services estimated that 21 million Americans have given up cigarette smoking. Surveys indicate that most smokers, up to 86 percent in one survey, say that they would like to break the habit.

Why do so many people want to stop smoking? Many have symptoms of diseases associated with smoking and have been ordered by their doctors to stop. Some want to stop because of the influence that their smoking has upon others, particularly

[1] This chapter is based largely upon the following: (1) Clifton R. Read, "If You Want to Give Up Cigarettes," American Cancer Society, 1968; (2) Dr. Daniel Horn and Dr. Donald T. Fredrickson, Reports to the World Conference on Smoking and Health, 1967; Dr. Borje Ejrup, "The Role of Nicotine in Smoking Pleasure"; Dr. Charles A. Ross, "Smoking Withdrawal Research Clinics," University of Arizona Press, 1967; Lois Mattox Miller, "The Dilemma of the Problem Smoker," Reader's Digest, May, 1964; and Patricia and Ron Deutsch, "Do You Really Want to Stop Smoking?" Reader's Digest, November, 1967.

children. Still others, although in good health, have decided that the health hazards and the costs of smoking are too great to justify the risk.

What are the rewards of stopping? Those who give up smoking have less illness, less hospitalization, less loss of time from work. Unless cancer has already started, discontinuance of cigarette smoking can mean longer life. Death rates of those who stop smoking decrease sharply as compared with those who continue smoking. Ten years after one has given up cigarette smoking his life expectancy is almost the same as for those who have never smoked regularly. Convincing evidence of the value of giving up smoking is that over a ten-year period the death rate from lung cancer among British physicians, a substantial portion of whom had stopped smoking, *decreased* by 30 percent while the death rate from lung cancer among British men in general *increased* by 25 percent.

Dr. Donald Fredrickson, Director of New York City's Smoking Control Program, says that a major reason that smokers decide to give up the habit is the evidence that by quitting smoking they can lower the chances of early disability—even during their thirties and forties. This is of particular concern to young smokers who are starting their careers and have or expect to have family and community responsibilities. Many smokers, Dr. Fredrickson adds, say: "Dying doesn't bother me—after all, once you're dead, you're dead. And I calculate my chances of developing lung cancer to be relatively small. But the idea of spending 15 or 20 years with a chronic disease that interferes with the enjoyment of life and reduces my ability to function well, that's too much. Smoking just isn't worth it!" [2]

These are long-range benefits: immediate rewards are reduction and early disappearance of cough, nasal stuffiness, and discharge; food tastes better, tensions decrease, sleep is sounder. Fatigue,

[2] "Diseases of the Chest," vol. 54, No. 3, p. 196, September, 1968.

shortness of breath, and that "dark brown" taste and "fuzzy feeling" in the mouth disappear. (For case histories of "Some Who Make It," see Appendix D.)

TYPES OF SMOKERS

Many smokers find it relatively easy to stop smoking if they *really* want to do so. Others find it difficult; almost unbearable for days, weeks, or even longer. To find the reasons for such differences psychologists have been studying the characteristics of smokers and conclude there are several types that may be classified somewhat as follows: stimulation smokers, handling smokers, relaxation smokers, crutch smokers, craving smokers, and habit smokers.[3] While the reasons given by people for smoking may in many cases overlap several of these classifications, one reason tends to be more prominent than the others. Psychologists believe that an analysis of one's smoking habits—even a self-analysis—is helpful in understanding the reasons and in breaking the habit. The Columbia Broadcasting System's National Smoking Test of 1968 was intended to aid in such a self-analysis.

Dr. Daniel Horn, Director of the U.S. Public Health Service Clearinghouse for Smoking and Health, who cooperated with CBS in the development of this test, explains these groupings as follows:

> *Stimulation smokers* smoke to give themselves a lift, to perk themselves up, to keep from slowing down. An example of the person who smokes for stimulation is the smoker who doesn't begin to live in the morning until he has had at least one cigarette at breakfast. Anyone in this "stimulation" group who wants to give up smoking will have to find some other

[3] Silvan Tomkins, director, Center for Research in Cognition and Affect, City University of New York; Daniel Horn, director, and Selwyn M. Waingrow, assistant to the director, National Clearinghouse for Smoking and Health, U.S. Public Health Service, Washington.

way of getting this kind of stimulation if he feels he needs it that much. Some stimulating activities such as eating and drinking can create problems of their own if you overdo them.

Handling smokers get gratification from having something to hold, something to manipulate, or something to watch, such as the exhaling of the smoke. Handling is a satisfaction for many pipe smokers who get most of their enjoyment from the feel of the pipe and the ritual they go through to keep it going. For smokers who get this kind of pleasure from cigarettes, rolling a pencil between the fingers often works just as well as a cigarette. Doodling is another form of the same kind of behavior.

Relaxation smokers enjoy smoking most when they are relaxed and comfortable. This is a favorite advertising theme: like the traditional cigar smoker who sits back after a good meal, and smokes a cigar to add to the pleasure he already feels. Most people who are "relaxation smokers" find they can get along quite easily without cigarettes.

Crutch smokers light cigarettes in moments of stress when they feel angry or upset or blue and want to take their minds off cares and worries. This kind of smoker may find it easy enough to quit cigarettes during a calm period, but hard to stay off them because the next personal crisis may result in lighting up again.

Craving smokers are psychologically addicted to cigarettes. A craving for the next cigarette begins to build up the moment they put out the last one. For this kind of smoker, the indications are that he must quit completely, all at once. It's called "going cold turkey." Tapering off is not likely to work for this person, because each cigarette starts the cycle of craving for the next cigarette.

There are marked differences between the so-called psychological addiction to tobacco and the addiction to certain drugs, the withdrawal of which results in acute illness and suffering.

Research so far indicates that the body's physical demand for the chemicals in cigarette smoke is probably less important than the psychological demand that builds up. The psychological addict cannot wait until breakfast time and often will light up before his feet hit the floor in the morning. He constantly thinks ahead to make sure there are enough cigarettes around to fill his need in the morning before he even goes to bed at night.

Quitting smoking is very difficult for this person. It is most important to get past the point of overwhelming craving for a cigarette. To do so it is often helpful to smoke far more cigarettes than usual for a short period, so that the taste for them becomes jaded, and then to isolate yourself completely from cigarettes. Once this kind of smoker quits cigarettes, he is apt to stay off for good.

Habit smokers smoke automatically: sometimes without being aware that they are smoking; they may find cigarettes in their mouths without remembering that they put them there; they frequently light a cigarette without realizing they have one still burning in the ashtray. These smokers no longer get much satisfaction from cigarettes. In regard to stopping there are three points to make about the habit smoker. First, he usually finds it rather easy to quit if he really wants to. Second, he can be successful in cutting down gradually and does not have to cut out cigarettes all at once. And third, the key to success in giving up smoking is in making himself aware of each cigarette by asking himself, "Do I really want this cigarette?" He will be surprised to find that the answer is frequently "No."

AIDS IN GIVING UP SMOKING

Many people—probably at least half of all smokers—can give up smoking without great difficulty if they *really* want to do so. Just

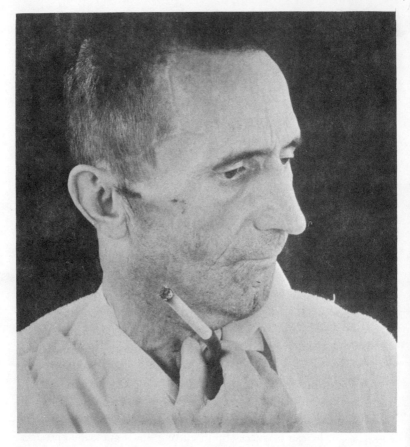

Figure 12.1. A *true addict: smoking through a tracheotomy tube after removal of the larynx because of cancer.* (*Courtesy Roswell Park Memorial Institute, Buffalo, N.Y.*)

wishing they could quit is not enough; they must be *determined* to quit. To develop determination one must have incentives, which requires an understanding of the rewards of stopping and of the seriousness of the health risks one assumes in continuing. The latter may come from information such as this book provides or from the development of symptoms and the advice of one's physician.

Programs to aid people who really want to give up smoking are of several types: (1) group sessions, often called withdrawal programs or clinics; (2) actual clinics operated by hospitals or medical or health organizations; (3) individual medical care provided by physicians in a doctor-patient relationship; (4) programs of self-help based upon books, pamphlets, magazine articles, radio or television programs, lectures, etc. (*Note:* See also Suggested Reference No. 17 in Appendix A, page 213.)

Group sessions

Group sessions conducted by various organizations reach large numbers of people and with proper leadership are helpful to many smokers. The Seventh-Day Adventist group has sponsored many such programs throughout the country. These are usually intensive programs on five consecutive evenings. The immediate results are good, but follow-up samplings indicate that a considerable proportion of those who stop resume the habit within a year.

An editor who worked with me on a revision on my book *Healthful Living* told me that she would like to give up smoking but was unable to do so and asked how she could get help. I told her of one of these programs that was to begin the next week. She attended regularly along with several hundred others in spite of the worst blizzard that New York City had had in years. She stopped smoking after the first session and did not smoke for more than a year. She told me later that she slipped back into the habit when she was having Christmas dinner with a brother and thought that on this occasion she would try "just one."

A modification of these group sessions has been developed by Dr. Donald Fredrickson of the New York City Health Department. The results of this program have been most encouraging: a follow-up of 200 participants several months after the completion of the program showed that 65 percent had stopped smoking, 15 percent had reduced their smoking by at least 75 percent, and 5 percent more had reduced their smoking by at least 50 percent.[4]

A distinguishing feature of Dr. Fredrickson's program is a staff of volunteer ex-smokers. Recruited from the program and drawn for the most part from the upper middle classes and the metropolitan business and professional world, these laymen function as group discussion leaders in the program's second and third phases. From a nucleus of thirteen, this volunteer staff grew, within ten months, to well over one hundred.

The program is conducted in three phases over an eight-month period. All sessions in Phase I and II are held in a local high school in mid-Manhattan. Phase III takes place on an impromptu basis in homes, offices, restaurants, etc.—wherever small groups can find a place to gather.

Phase I (orientation) This commences with an evening lecture delivered by a physician (the Program Director) and is immediately followed by seven days of "home work." Guided by printed instructions, the smoker initiates the process of (1) developing strong motivation, (2) bringing the habit to a fully conscious level, and (3) gaining insight into some of the psychological mechanisms supporting his smoking behavior.

The objective of the lecture is to convince the smoker (1) that he possesses the *capacity* to permanently free himself of the habit; (2) that the clinic has a therapy which, when applied according to instructions, is *highly effective*; and (3) that withdrawal has the potential for being an enriching and genuinely rewarding experience.

The instructional material from which the smoker works the first week consists of techniques borrowed from other experimental

[4] From report by Dr. Donald Fredrickson to the World Conference on Smoking and Health, September, 1967.

clinics. These include (1) developing a list of reasons for wanting to stop smoking—to assist the smoker in focusing his motivation; (2) keeping a careful daily smoking record (noting the time, the activities, and/or the feeling states associated with each cigarette) —to help break into the subconscious and reflex aspects of smoking; and (3) ranking cigarettes according to their relative importance in the daily routine (each cigarette is assigned a numbered category, 1 to 4, with each succeeding category containing cigarettes of lesser importance than those in the preceding one). This instruction is to aid the smoker in developing insights into some of the factors related to the maintenance of his cigarette habit.

Phase II (withdrawal) Smokers are placed in groups of 15 with two volunteer ex-smokers assigned to each. One ex-smoker serves as group moderator (discussion leader), the other as moderator-in-training. These groups meet twice a week for four weeks, then once a week for an additional four weeks. Meetings are held in the early evening and last approximately ninety minutes.

The groups are composed of approximately equal numbers of men and women, and are constructed to reflect two age categories; those under forty and those forty and over are placed in separate groups. Very heavy smokers—over three packs a day—are placed in separate groups. Friends who attend meetings are encouraged to work together in the same group.

Two basic approaches to withdrawal are offered: sudden ("cold turkey") and gradual. During the most recent program over 90 percent chose the gradual approach.

Once in a group smokers have three goals to accomplish: (1) assist each other in building a strong motivation, (2) constructively confront each other's attitudes, particularly those relating to events and feelings associated with the withdrawal experience itself, and

(3) provide mutual guidance and support during and immediately following the period of withdrawal. All meetings follow a standard format.

Sessions begin with smokers reporting on their progress (or lack thereof) since the last meeting. Each smoker's problems are presented in a "consultation session" where the group, through frank and open discussion, constructively discuss the difficulties being encountered in withdrawal. When all have reported, the group prepares for a "work period." In teams of four, formed during the first two sessions, the smoker develops a plan for the next step in his reduction program. Participants are instructed to commit themselves at each meeting to a program of reduction wherein they will maintain or increase their rate of smoking withdrawal. The exact amount and the "strategy" for this reduction are left to the smoker, working with his colleagues, to decide. The reduction pledge is entered on a smoking record card and the group reassembles. Each smoker, identifying himself with his team, announces his pledge to the entire group and a general discussion follows.

During the first three sessions, a small, part-time professional staff (three physicians, a clinical psychologist, and a public health social worker) circulate among the groups answering medical questions and assisting the moderators in identifying individuals with special problems. At the conclusion of every third meeting, participants are invited to join the program director for a general question and answer session. Meetings are supplemented with "fact sheets" on smoking and health and lists of suggestions ("Tip Sheets") on techniques that successful ex-smokers have found helpful in withstanding the urge to smoke.

Phase III (reinforcement)   With completion of Phase II, there is a regrouping in preparation for follow-up. Groups of 12 to 15 are structured with a moderator and moderator-in-training assigned to each. Meetings are spaced at increasing intervals, once a week for three to four weeks, then once every other week for five to six months, and are conducted at a time and location convenient to the group. Every conceivable kind of location—offices, homes, restaurants, bars—is utilized. Following each meeting the group reports to the program's central office by means of a large postal card on which is indicated the progress of each participant and the time and location of the next meeting. Once a month all participants are invited to join with the Program Director for a brief talk followed by a question and answer period.

The program's basic therapeutic ingredient is a form of group support mediated through lay-directed discussion and social interchange. The idea of a clinic conducted by laymen was borrowed from such "anonymous" organizations as Alcoholics Anonymous, Gamblers Anonymous, and Weight Watchers. The conceptual notion underlying this approach comes from certain ideas about mechanisms which lead to and support cigarette habituation.

Basically, the idea is that cigarette smoking, or rather the process of becoming habituated to cigarettes, involves an act of *learning*. With the "learning theory" concept as a cornerstone, the smoker is instructed that his primary task is to teach or retrain himself to be a nonsmoker. This is accomplished quite literally by retracing the steps he took in becoming a smoker. As with any other learning experience, the smoker is told that he will have to be highly motivated and faithfully exercise the cardinal virtues of patience and persistence. Above all he must practice his nonsmoking behavior. He must experience the many activities and feeling states formerly associated with smoking without the benefit of cigarettes.

Another assumption that has guided the development of the program is that three tasks, when undertaken currently, maximize one's chances for permanent smoking behavior change. These are (1) developing strong personal motivation characterized by a sense of immediacy, (2) commitment to a clearly defined program of action, and (3) identifying and confronting attitudes that resist behavior change.

The smoker's behavior is the principal focus of attack. The technique of having each individual determine his own rate and manner of reduction seems a fairly satisfactory solution to the difficult problem of designing individual cessation strategies and has proven effective in maintaining the smoker's withdrawal momentum. In working with the group, the only "rule" that all follow is to maintain or increase this rate from one meeting to the next. Gradual withdrawal is explained as a "means to an end," a way of bringing the smoker into meaningful involvement with the program so as to psychologically prepare him for the time when he will make a complete break with his cigarettes.

For many, permanent smoking cessation undoubtedly requires some type of long-term reinforcement of nonsmoking behavior. Dr. Fredrickson says that his present format is designed to provide at least a limited kind of extended reinforcement. All participants are invited to join follow-up groups at the conclusion of Phase II. The most meaningful reinforcement comes, however, to those ex-smokers who accept assignments as volunteer staff. As soon as one stops smoking, he qualifies for and is invited to accept a staff position. The majority serve as group Moderators, Alternates, or Trainees, though other assignments are available (clerical, etc.). Smokers understand that in accepting responsibility for helping others break the habit, they will bring into play a highly effective means of reinforcing their own nonsmoking behavior.

Nonsmoking and cessation-of-smoking programs are creating a great and increasing interest throughout the United States. Thousands of persons who have heard of them have asked to be enrolled for the next one. Results to date have been most encouraging, but Dr. Fredrickson considers the program still in an experimental and developmental stage.[5]

[5] Requests for further information about the program may be addressed to: Dr. Donald T. Fredrickson, New York City Department of Health, 125 Worth Street, New York, N.Y. 10013.

Smoking withdrawal clinics

Several smoking withdrawal clinics have been operated on an experimental basis by New York State's Roswell Park Memorial (Cancer) Institute in Buffalo. The subjects were all volunteers from the community, of whom 100 out of 1,500 applicants were accepted for the first program. The programs involved both group sessions held once weekly for four consecutive weeks and out-patient clinic conferences and treatments. Approximately 35 percent immediately stopped smoking and over the long term about 20 percent gave up cigarettes. Other conclusions were that an appreciation of the relationship between cigarette smoking and disease appeared to be the most significant factor relating to successful withdrawal and that those who are the most stable emotionally are the ones most successful in giving up cigarettes.

Personalized medical treatment

Individual medical attention seems to be necessary for many "addicted" hard-core smokers. The physician who has had the most extensive experience in treating smokers in a doctor-patient relationship is Dr. Borge Ejrup of the New York Hospital–Cornell Medical Center, formerly of the Karolinska Institute in Stockholm. In 1955 Dr. Ejrup opened the first of six withdrawal clinics in Stockholm. His medical specialty is cardiovascular diseases. He became interested in the smoking problem when he told patients with heart disease that they must stop smoking and their usual reply was "I would like to, but how?"

Dr. Ejrup's treatment program usually consists of an initial phase of daily visits five days a week for two weeks, followed by a tapering-off schedule that may extend over a period up to two years. If necessary, daily injections of lobeline hydrochloride—a nicotine-like substance—are given during the first two weeks. In addition to the administration of lobeline, the treatment includes counseling, special exercises, advice concerning diet, and, for some patients in whom tension or irritability develops, sedatives and tranquilizers.

Of more than a thousand persons treated in Sweden, over 75 percent stopped smoking entirely during treatment and another 22 percent reduced their smoking to less than one-fourth of their previous consumption. In a relatively small number of long-time smokers at the New York Hospital clinic, 61 percent stopped entirely and 29 percent cut down to less than one-fourth the number of cigarettes they had smoked before.

Hypnosis seems to help some people to give up smoking but does not help others. If one is considering hypnosis, he should discuss it with his physician.

Quitting on your own [6]

Self-help or do-it-yourself programs are all that many smokers need. Sufficiently motivated individuals are convinced that they can manage their own lives. They enjoy challenging themselves; with the exercise of willpower they break the habit. The ex-smoker teaches himself a more positive, more constructive, more rewarding behavior.

To think of giving up cigarettes as a denial is a mistake. The smoker should not feel that he is giving up something of value. If he does, he will feel sorry for himself; he will brood on his sufferings, which will become increasingly severe and possibly unendurable. Instead he should feel that he is adding something to his life—a new dimension of self-control. He is teaching himself a more positive, constructive, self-fulfilling way to behave. There is

---

[6] For more specific suggestions on how to break the cigarette habit, see Clifton R. Read's American Cancer Society publication, "If You Want to Give Up Cigarettes," presented here as Appendix D, p. 231. (See also ref. p. 142.)

evidence that the development of control over cigarette smoking, for some at least, tends to influence other areas of behavior, bringing a renewed sense of one's ability and possibly even an actual increase in one's capacity to deal more constructively with other "problems of living." When experienced, this can serve as a powerful incentive reinforcing nonsmoking behavior.

Some smokers, often successful in other aspects of living, find that willpower does not enable them to give up cigarettes. They try to stop; they do not succeed; and they feel guilty about their failure. This does not indicate that they are weak, merely different. Their approach must be less through determination and more through learning new behavior and through perseverance.

Some tips that may help

A good book or pamphlet on the subject may help.

Placing cigarettes in unaccustomed places or pockets and putting matches, lighters, and ashtrays out of reach help to break the unconscious routine.

Drinking frequent glasses of water; changing from coffee to tea if coffee has been a signal for a cigarette; nibbling fruit, crackers, cookies, sucking hard candies or chewing gum or bits of ginger are helpful to many.

Keeping away for a few days from friends who are smokers or working in the library or other rooms where smoking is forbidden may reduce the temptation to smoke.

Deep breathing, a walk around the block, or other, more strenuous exercise relieves tension.

Bantron or Nikoban tablets are recommended by some doctors, not by others. One should check with his physician to make sure there is no medical reason for not using them.

Most persons select a day on which they will quit absolutely; others find it easier to reduce gradually. To reduce gradually one must formulate a definite schedule: decide not to smoke between nine and ten, eleven and twelve, one and three; increase the no-smoking periods from an hour to an hour and a half, then to two hours; smoke only after meals; smoke only in the evening. Or it may help to give up smoking first at the times that smoking means least to you, i.e., during relatively low-tension, low-pressure periods, and gradually extend this to other times of the day.

In gradual withdrawal you can wrap your cigarettes in many sheets of paper, or strive to use only the left hand if normally the right hand held the cigarette, or hold the cigarette in a different corner of your mouth. You can smoke only half of each cigarette, or can make it a point not to have the change necessary to purchase cigarettes from a machine.

Many people decide to stop for only one day at a time. They promise themselves 24 hours of freedom from cigarettes. Then when the day is over they make a pledge to desist for another day; then another, and another. At the end of any 24-hour period they can go back to cigarettes without betraying themselves—but they usually do not.

When you have saved a bit of money by not buying cigarettes, treat yourself to a good dinner, a good play, a new record, or something that you or your family will appreciate. A physician friend who used to smoke three packs a day rewarded himself and his family with a new television set at the end of the first year that he had "been off" cigarettes. That was five years ago and he has continued these annual rewards ever since.

Increasingly, health departments, health centers, hospitals, and individual physicians are offering help to cigarette smokers who wish to get rid of the habit.

At the World Conference on Smoking and Health in September, 1967, Sir George Godber said: "It is never *too late* to stop smoking for the benefit of one's health; and it is never *too early* to stop for the benefit of those—particularly children—who will be influenced by your example."

GOVERNMENT RESPONSIBILITY

CHAPTER THIRTEEN

An important responsibility of government is to protect the health of the people. Some of this responsibility rests with the federal government, some with state governments, and some with local governmental units. In regard to a health hazard of such magnitude as cigarette smoking, one wonders why government has not done more about it. The reasons for this are many and complex.

Before the harmful effects of cigarette smoking were recognized, the tobacco industry had grown into one of the largest, most powerful businesses in the country. Farmers profited from the raising of tobacco; manufacturers from its processing and distribution; public relations firms from its promotion; newspapers, magazines, radio, and television from its advertising; retail merchants and vending machines from its sale; charitable, youth-serving, education and research organizations from its grants and subsidies;

and government of all levels from taxes both upon the industry and upon the many millions of purchasers of tobacco products.

Some regulation of cigarette smoking was intended by states which many years ago passed laws to prohibit the sale of cigarettes to persons below a specified age ranging from fifteen to twenty-one. Forty-seven out of fifty states have laws of this type on their books. Only Georgia and Louisiana never had such laws; Wisconsin repealed its law as unenforceable. These laws, however, were rarely enforced and were completely ignored when vending machines began to dispense cigarettes. This was modified somewhat later when the National Automatic Merchandizing Association directed that stickers be affixed to vending machines stating that the sale of cigarettes to minors is illegal wherever laws of this type exist. Local laws or ordinances also prohibit smoking in certain places, such as stores, theaters, and subways, but these restrictions are in the interest of fire prevention rather than of health.

The executive agency of the federal government with primary responsibility for health is the U.S. Public Health Service. Although evidence of the relationship of cigarette smoking to various diseases had been accumulating since the early 1950s, the first statement from the Public Health Service on the subject was made by its Surgeon General, Leroy F. Burney, M.D., in the *Journal of the American Medical Association* in November, 1959. The heart of this statement was that "the weight of evidence at present implicates smoking as the principal etiological factor in the increased incidence of lung cancer."

THE SURGEON GENERAL'S ADVISORY COMMITTEE

In June, 1961, the American Cancer Society, the American Heart Association, the American Public Health Association and the National Tuberculosis and Respiratory Disease Association jointly requested President John F. Kennedy "to appoint a Commission to consider the responsibilities of government, of business and of voluntary agencies relative to the health hazards of cigarette smoking and to recommend a solution of this health problem that would protect the public and would interfere least with the freedom of industry and the happiness of individuals."

On June 7, 1962, the then Surgeon General, Dr. Luther Terry, announced, with the approval of the President, that he was establishing an "expert committee to undertake a comprehensive review of all data on smoking and health." The members of this committee were respected scientists who had previously expressed no opinion about the relationship of tobacco to health. All members were approved for appointment by the tobacco industry as well as by the American Medical Association and several national health agencies. Half of the committee members were cigarette smokers. (For list of members see page 229.)

On January 11, 1964, after some 15 months of intensive study, this Advisory Committee to the Surgeon General issued its monumental unanimous report stating that "cigarette smoking is a health hazard of sufficient importance in the United States to warrant appropriate remedial action." The committee stated unequivocally that "cigarette smoking is causally related to lung cancer in men; the magnitude of the effect of cigarette smoking far outweighs other factors. The data for women, though less extensive, point in the same direction." Air pollution was found to be a very minor factor in the cause of the disease, far outweighed by cigarette smoking.

The death rate from heart disease, the report noted, is 70 percent higher in cigarette smokers than in nonsmokers, and although there was not enough evidence to say positively that smoking causes heart disease, there was enough to assume that it is a cause and to take action against it.

Another conclusion of great importance was that "cigarette smoking is the most important of the causes of chronic bronchitis in the United States and increases the risk of dying from chronic bronchitis and emphysema."

The report analyzed the statistical, pathological, clinical, and experimental evidence in relation to smoking and other diseases. A total of more than 4,000 published reports were studied and more than 150 investigators personally interviewed. The result was the most comprehensive and authoritative report on this subject ever made.[1]

NATIONAL CLEARINGHOUSE FOR SMOKING AND HEALTH

Following this report the Public Health Service established the National Clearinghouse for Smoking and Health "to disseminate information on this subject, to conduct studies and to stimulate control measures." Congress has appropriated $2 million a year for this program—less than half the amount it provides each year for research on how to produce more and better tobacco.

The Cigarette Labeling and Advertising Act of 1965 requires that the Secretary of Health, Education, and Welfare (of which the U.S. Public Health Service is one unit) shall report to Congress by July 1, 1967 and annually thereafter any new further information on the health consequences of smoking, together with any legislative recommendations he may wish to make. Pursuant to this directive, in 1967 a report on "The Health Consequences of Smoking" was prepared by the Clearinghouse on Smoking and Health and was transmitted by Dr. William A. Stewart, the Surgeon Gen-

[1] "Smoking and Health, Report of the Advisory Committee to the Surgeon General of the Public Health Service," U.S. Department of Health, Education, and Welfare, Washington, Public Health Service Publication 1103, 1964.

eral of the Public Health Service, to the Secretary of Health, Education, and Welfare and to the Congress.

This 200-page report reviews more than 2,000 research studies published since the 1964 report and concludes that these additional studies confirm and strengthen the conclusion that "cigarette smoking is a health hazard of sufficient importance in the United States to warrant appropriate remedial action." This review goes beyond the original report in that it summarizes new and significant studies of the relation of smoking to illness and disability as well as to premature death.

On July 1, 1968, a second follow-up report was submitted to Congress by the Public Health Service. This report presents even more conclusive evidence than the earlier reports that cigarette smoking is a major causative factor of coronary heart disease and of emphysema. The report also contains recommendations by the Secretary of Health, Education, and Welfare for the reduction of this health hazard.

THE FEDERAL TRADE COMMISSION'S RESPONSIBILITY

Another agency of government involved with the smoking prob lem is the Federal Trade Commission. This commission was established to protect the consuming public from false, misleading, deceptive, or unfair advertising (including labeling) of products that may endanger human health or safety.

After the release of the Surgeon's General's Report on Smoking and Health the Federal Trade Commission concluded that cigarette advertising was deceptive (misleading) and that the commission had a responsibility to warn the public of the health hazards of cigarette smoking. To accomplish this it proposed that cigarette packages state the amount of tar and nicotine in the smoke of the cigarette which the package contains and that cigarette packages and cigarette advertising carry a statement such as: "Caution: Cigarette Smoking Is Dangerous to Health. It May Cause Death from Cancer and Other Diseases."

This warning was to be required on cigarette packages beginning January 1, 1965, and in cigarette advertising beginning July 1, 1965. The tobacco industry first obtained a postponement of the effective dates of this ruling and then prevailed upon Congress to negate the ruling by passing the Cigarette Labeling and Advertising Act, which requires that all packages of cigarettes sold in this country must carry the label "Cigarette Smoking May Be Hazardous to Your Health," but prohibits the Federal Trade Commission and state and local governments from requiring any other label on cigarette packages and any warnings in cigarette advertising at least until 1969.

Although this act prevented any requirement that tar and nicotine content be indicated on cigarette packages, the Federal Trade Commission did establish a laboratory to determine the tar and nicotine content of the smoke of cigarettes on the American market, and it is making the results of these tests available periodically to the public.

The Cigarette Labeling and Advertising Act also required that about July 1, 1967 and annually thereafter the Federal Trade Commission report to Congress concerning the effectiveness of the warning label, and upon current practices of cigarette advertising and promotion, with "recommendations for legislation that are deemed appropriate."

After an intensive study the Federal Trade Commission made a detailed report to Congress with the following summary and recommendations:

The Commission believes that the warning label on cigarette packages has not succeeded in overcoming the prevalent attitude toward cigarette smoking created and maintained by the cigarette companies through their advertisements, particularly the barrage of commercials on television, which portray smoking as a harmless and enjoyable social activity that is not habit forming and involves no hazards to health.

It appears to the Commission, from the switch toward filter cigarettes and the popularity of low tar and nicotine cigarettes, that a substantial segment of the public is most concerned about the health hazards of cigarette smoking. Many smokers would like to give up the habit, but don't and won't. Some of these have switched to brands that they believe, often erroneously, to be less hazardous. The Commission favors giving smokers as much information about the risks involved in smoking as is possible and to that end favors mandatory disclosure of tar and nicotine content, as measured by a standard test. Until this is done, millions of smokers will continue to be deceived by false claims of "mildness" and misleading portrayals of filters.

Non-cigarette smokers, particularly the teenagers who constitute an ever-increasing class of potential customers, seem in large part to have been unaffected by the warning on the package alone. The cigarette advertisements, especially on television and radio, that are more frequently viewed and heard by teenagers than other segments of the population, have been successful in their subtle but effective attempts to persuade teenagers to smoke despite the known health hazards. To protect this group the Commission feels it imperative that adequate health warnings be included in all cigarette advertising.

Cigarette smoking today poses a very great but preventable public health menace. It is strongly habituating, and habitual smokers subject themselves to a number of debilitating illnesses and early death. Despite this, cigarette companies have spent billions of dollars (in 1966 almost $300 million) on inducing the people to take up this habit so dangerous to health. In the interest of fairness to the adults of tomorrow, advertising without an adequate warning should not be permitted to continue. Self-regulation by the industry has proved to be ineffectual.

Cigarette commercials continue to appeal to youth and continue to blot out any consciousness of the health hazards. Cigarette advertisements continue to appear on programs watched and heard repeatedly by millions of teenagers. Today, teenagers are constantly exposed to an endless barrage of subtle messages that cigarette smoking increases popularity, makes one more masculine or attractive to the opposite sex, enhances one's social poise, etc. To allow the American people, and expecially teenagers, the opportunity to make an informed and deliberate choice of whether or not to start smoking, they must be freed from constant exposure to such one-sided blandishments and told the whole story.

Recommendations. The Commission believes that legislation accomplishing the following objectives is necessary:

1 Section 4 of the Federal Cigarette Labeling and Advertising Act should be amended by changing the required warning statement to read: "Warning: Cigarette Smoking Is Dangerous to Health and May Cause Death from Cancer and Other Diseases."

2 The warning statement should be required to appear in all advertisements as well as on all cigarette packages;

3 A statement setting forth the tar and nicotine content of each cigarette should be required to appear on the package and in all cigarette advertising;

4 Cigarette advertising on television and radio should be barred entirely. Alternately, cigarette advertising on television and

radio should be limited as to hours in which it may appear; the extent to which it may appear; and the types of programs on which it may appear.[2]

5 Increased appropriations should be made to the Department of Health, Education, and Welfare for education of the public (especially young people) as to the health hazards of smoking;

6 Appropriations should be made for research under the direction of the National Institutes of Health on the development of less hazardous cigarettes.

CONGRESSIONAL ACTION

The ultimate responsibility within the federal government for health measures rests with Congress. Government departments, commissions, and agencies can act only within the authority given them by Congress. As noted earlier, the health hazards of cigarette smoking were first considered by Congress in 1965 after the Federal Trade Commission proposed that warning labels on cigarette packages and in cigarette advertising be required. The resulting legislation was the Cigarette Labeling and Advertising Act of 1965.

A New York Times editorial called this law "a shocking piece of special-interest legislation—a bill to protect the economic health of the tobacco industry by freeing it of proper regulation." [3] An article in the Atlantic Monthly [4] described the political maneuvering behind this legislation under the title "The Quiet Victory of the Cigarette Lobby: How It Found the Best Filter Yet—

---

[2] The fourth recommendation did not appear, as did the others, in the 1967 report; it was not presented to Congress until 1968.

[3] New York Times, July 9, 1965.

[4] Elizabeth B. Drew, "The Quiet Victory of the Cigarette Lobby: How It Found the Best Filter Yet—Congress," Atlantic Monthly, vol. 216, p. 76, September, 1965.

Congress." The reason for this title is that the tobacco industry got from Congress the type of law that it wanted.[5]

Reported reasons for this legislation were that the public concern which followed publication of the Surgeon General's Report on Smoking and Health and the pending FTC regulations for warnings on cigarette packages and in cigarette advertising convinced the tobacco industry that some action by Congress was inevitable. In order that it interfere as little as possible with "business as usual," the industry decided to accept a weak label on cigarette packages provided that the legislation would prevent any regulation of cigarette advertising. This was accomplished by inserting into the proposed law a provision that took from the FTC and all state or local governments their authority to require any warning on cigarette packages other than the one approved by Congress and also prevented any warnings in cigarette advertising.

The tactics of the tobacco industry in connection with this legislation were a masterpiece of strategy and lobbying. At House and Senate committee hearings, committee members friendly to the industry attempted to discredit both the Surgeon General's Report and the testimony given by the Surgeon General, the Chairman of the Federal Trade Commission, and the representatives of various medical and health organizations. The tobacco industry then presented a number of physicians who testified that they disagreed with the conclusions of the Surgeon General's Advisory Committee and that in their opinion there was no real evidence that cigarette smoking is harmful.

That the significance of these testimonies was understood by at least some members of Congress is evident from the report of the Senate Commerce Committee, which had conducted the Senate hearings on this proposed legislation. This report said in part:

[5] Lois Mattox Miller and James Monahan, "To the Cigarette Makers: Just the Facts Please," Reader's Digest, November, 1966.

While there remain a substantial number of individual physicians and scientists—the Commerce Committee received
testimony from 39 of them—who do not believe that it has
been demonstrated scientifically that smoking causes cancer or
other diseases, no prominent medical or scientific body under-
taking a scientific review of the evidence has reached conclusions opposed to those of the Surgeon General's Advisory
Committee.—The Commerce Committee, therefore, concurs
in the judgment that "appropriate remedial action" is war-
ranted.

This testimony of the tobacco industry's witnesses, however, provided some rationalization or excuse for the Congressmen and
Senators who voted for the bill promoted by the industry. These
statements have been useful also to the public relations activities
of the cigarette industry.

THE FEDERAL COMMUNICATIONS COMMISSION

Another government agency that has become concerned with cigarette advertising is the Federal Communications Commission. It is
the responsibility of this commission to see to it that the airways,
which belong to the public, are used in the public interest. Concerning this the Honorable William E. Henry, Chairman of the
Federal Communications Commission in 1966, said in an address
before the National Association of Broadcasters:

From the advertising presently being carried on radio and
television no one would ever know that the great bulk of
medical opinion, including a Surgeon General's Report, has
concluded that there is an adverse causal relationship between
cigarette smoking and health. Nor is there the slightest hint
that the Congress of the United States last year passed a
Cigarette Labeling Act which requires every pack to contain

the warning—and I quote—"Caution: Cigarette Smoking May Be Hazardous to Your Health."

Despite all of this, the sign on broadcasting's door for cigarette advertisers reads: "Business as usual."

A startling anomaly is thus created. Television viewers in particular are led to believe that cigarette smoking is the key to fun and games with the opposite sex, good times at home and abroad, social success and virility. But as the individual approaches the tobacco stand and mystically changes from television viewer to cigarette customer, so the message changes. Life with cigarettes is no longer beautiful: the package warns that smoking may have ugly consequences indeed.

A year later the Communications Commission decided that it was not in the public interest for the airways to be used by radio and television to advertise cigarettes without warnings of the health hazards involved in smoking. The commission therefore ruled that radio and television stations which advertise cigarettes must give health agencies a "reasonable" amount of time to present information concerning the health damage caused by smoking. As a result of this ruling, many television and radio stations are running spot announcements about the hazards of smoking. The ruling, however, is being attacked in the courts by the broadcasting and tobacco industries.

FUTURE LEGISLATION

Both the U.S. Public Health Service and the Federal Trade Commission have annually reported findings to Congress since passage of the cigarette labeling law. Several bills have been introduced in Congress consistent with the conclusions and the recommendations of these two reports.

Some state and local governments may consider action to regulate the promotion and sale of cigarettes when the restrictions contained in the federal law expire.

What new legislation will be enacted or changes made in the 1965 law when the present law expires in 1969, only time will tell. However, in view of the tremendous influence of the tobacco industry, and of radio, television, newspapers, magazines, merchants, and other groups that profit from the promotion or sale of cigarettes, it is unlikely that any substantial changes will be made unless and until the public is really concerned and until voters "back home" tell their Congressmen and Senators in Washington what they think and what they want done about it. A silent unorganized majority is powerless against a highly organized special interest group.

EFFORTS TO REDUCE SMOKING

CHAPTER FOURTEEN

The use of tobacco has long been opposed by the Mormons, the Seventh-Day Adventists, and certain other religious groups. In the last century most states enacted laws prohibiting the sale of cigarettes to persons below specified ages. These laws were mostly ignored, but in the 1890s the women's clubs of Chicago clamored for legislation to curb tobacco sales. This went unheeded until "Bathhouse John" (Coughlin), the notorious political boss of Chicago's infamous First Ward, made a dramatic move for action. To the surprise of everyone he introduced into the City Council a measure requiring an excise fee of $100 for all shops selling cigarettes and barring their sale entirely within 200 yards of schools. "Bathhouse John" presumably did this to improve his political image and quiet some of the violent criticism of him and his associates. The "Tobacco Trust" railed against it, but the Council passed the statute. Concerning it the *Chicago Tribune* commented editorially: "By this measure he (Coughlin) will drive from the school areas the petty peddlers in death who have been inviting the children to ruin." [1]

For many years some physicians have been advising against the use of tobacco. It was not, however, until after the reports in 1954 and 1957 of the American Cancer Society's first prospective study that there was any organized effort to inform the public of the hazards of cigarette smoking. In 1960 the Board of Directors of the Cancer Society stated that "cigarette smoking is the major cause of lung cancer" and authorized "widespread dissemination of information concerning this to physicians and the public with primary initial emphasis on teenagers." *Reader's Digest* has cooperated fully and since 1954 has published 15 articles on the subject by Roving Editor Lois Mattox Miller and Senior Editor James Monahan. In addition, the *Digest* has published more than 50 articles on this subject by other authors.

THE MEDICAL BULLETIN ON TOBACCO

Because of increasing evidence that cigarette smoking contributes to coronary heart disease, chronic bronchitis, and emphysema as well as lung cancer, the American Heart Association, the National Tuberculosis and Respiratory Disease Association, and the American Public Health Association became concerned about cigarette smoking and joined with the American Cancer Society in the publication of the *Medical Bulletin on Tobacco*. The purpose of this quarterly publication has been to bring to the attention of physicians and other readers summaries of significant new information concerning the effects of tobacco on health. Initially the *Bulletin* was mailed to all physicians in the United States; later to all dentists and to some nurses and other public health workers.

---

[1] Lloyd Wendt and Herman Hogan, "Bosses in Lusty Chicago—The Story of Bathhouse John and Hinky Dink," Indiana University Press, Bloomington, Ind., 1967.

These four national voluntary health organizations also joined in writing a letter to President John F. Kennedy urging him to evaluate the health hazards of cigarette smoking and to recommend remedial action. This resulted in the appointment of the Surgeon General's Advisory Committee on Smoking and Health. (See pages 154 and 229.)

INTERAGENCY COUNCIL ON SMOKING AND HEALTH

Following the release of the report of this committee the Surgeon General, Luther Terry, called a conference of representatives of the major health organizations concerned with the problem to consider what might be done to reduce the hazards so convincingly documented by this report. This led to further conferences and finally to the organization of the National Interagency Council on Smoking and Health. The purpose of this Council is (1) to use its professional talents to bring to the nation—particularly to the young—an increasing awareness of the harmfulness of cigarette smoking; (2) to encourage, support and assist national, state and local smoking and health programs; and (3) to generate and coordinate public interest and action related to this area of health.

The current membership of the council consists of 25 national organizations and five government agencies.[2] The membership of this council is shown in Table 14.1. The council's very modest budget is provided by voluntary contributions of member organizations.

State interagency committees or councils were established in California and in one or two other states prior to the organization of the National Council. Today interagency councils are operative in

[2] The author of this book served as a member of the organizing committee of this council and as its vice-chairman from 1965 to 1968.

40 states and in many cities throughout the country. The primary function of these councils is to coordinate and stimulate action by member groups rather than to operate programs of their own.

TABLE 14.1 National Interagency Council on Smoking and Health

Council membership at the beginning of 1969 consisted of the following professional, private, voluntary, and governmental organizations:

Active Members	American Academy of Pediatrics
	American Association for Health, Physical Education and Recreation
	American Association of School Administrators
	American Cancer Society
	American College Health Association
	American College of Chest Physicians
	American College of Physicians
	American College of Surgeons
	American Dental Association
	American Heart Association
	American Hospital Association
	American Nurses Association
	American Pharmaceutical Association
	American Public Health Association
	American School Health Association
	Association of Classroom Teachers
	Association of State and Territorial Health Officers
	National Congress of Parents and Teachers
	National League for Nursing
	National Tuberculosis and Respiratory Disease Association
	U.S. Children's Bureau
	U.S. Department of Defense
	U.S. Office of Education
	U.S. Public Health Service
	U.S. Veterans Administration
Affiliate Members	Boys' Clubs of America
	National Board of Young Men's Christian Association
	National Board of Young Women's Christian Association
	National Student Nurses' Association
	Public Health Cancer Association of America
Officers	Luther L. Terry, M.D.—Chairman
	Sol R. Baker, M.D.—Vice-Chairman
	Daniel Horn, Ph.D.—Secretary
Members at Large	Emerson Foote
	Luther L. Terry, M.D.

The National Interagency Council testified before Congress on the cigarette-labeling bills and arranged for testimony at these hearings by representatives of member organizations. It also sponsored the World Conference on Smoking and Health under the management of the American Cancer Society.

VOLUNTARY HEALTH AGENCIES

Members of the National Interagency Council, notably the American Cancer Society, the American Heart Association, the National Tuberculosis and Respiratory Disease Association, the National Congress of Parents and Teachers, the U.S. Public Health Service, and the U.S. Children's Bureau, have greatly expanded their public information and professional and public education programs on smoking and health. In fact, the National Congress of Parents and Teachers with the support of the National Clearinghouse for Smoking and Health is sponsoring and stimulating a nationwide program of instruction in public schools on the health hazards of cigarette smoking.

Voluntary national organizations are providing television and radio programs and spot announcements about cigarette smoking. Motion pictures, posters, pamphlets, and other educational materials are produced and distributed by these organizations, by the U.S. Public Health Service, by the U.S. Children's Bureau, and by state and local health departments.

THE SOCIAL ACCEPTABILITY OF SMOKING

Efforts to reduce smoking are faced with the difficult problem of how to reduce its appeal and its social acceptability. As the Federal Trade Commission states, cigarette advertisements still portray smoking, to both children and adults, "as a harmless and enjoyable social activity that is not habit forming and involves no hazard to health." [3]

''Federal Trade Commission Report to Congress on the Cigarette Advertising Act.'' June 30, 1967, p. 28.

The ashtrays and matches in every restaurant and hotel room, in many public buildings, hospital lobbies, doctors' offices, and private homes, are both a symbol of the acceptability of smoking and an encouragement to smoke.

Also, as Dr. Borje Ejrup, Director of the Anti-Smoking Clinic of the New York Hospital–Cornell Medical Center, writes: [4]

> The complications of modern life may encourage smoking as a specific behaviour. Those with no creative talents substitute smoking for their passivity, others, tortured by loneliness, find the cigarette or pipe a good companion. Still others use the cigarette as a tool rather than a drug to promote sociability. Making friends is easier when one has something to offer, to take, to discuss—a mutual behaviour. [It makes] young people . . . feel mature to belong to a group rather than to be set aside as too young. To do as others do gives them a warm feeling and helps eliminate shyness. They do not expect too much and they know, or will soon discover, that the physiological effect of smoking in the beginning is not a pleasant one.

> Of the many other factors determining why and how much a person smokes and which smoking pattern he prefers, the *environmental influences* are of great importance, especially in regulating the amount of tobacco smoked. It seems not to be the general or local nicotine effect that determines the number of cigarettes in the following examples from the tobacco withdrawal clinics:

> **Example 1** A 50-year-old female office worker was not permitted to smoke while working. She started smoking at age 30 and was entirely satisfied with 4–5 cigarettes daily for 15 years. After that time office regulations were changed

⁴ Borje Ejrup, ''The Role of Nicotine in Smoking Pleasure, Nicotinism, Treatment, Tobacco Alkaloids and Related Compounds,'' Proceedings of the Fourth International Symposium, Stockholm, February 1964, Permagon Press, New York, 1965.

to permit smoking during working hours. The number of cigarettes smoked rapidly rose to 20 a day. This distressed her as she felt the old regime was more conducive to well-being. On the 20-a-day regime she acquired chronic bronchitis, fatigue and shortness of breath. After clinic attendance she was able to stop smoking entirely.

In this case the environment was the direct cause of increase in the amount of tobacco smoked rather than a need or craving for nicotine.

Example 2 A 32-year-old sailor wished to eliminate smoking entirely because of health and economic reasons. For many years he found satisfaction in smoking 20 cigarettes daily at home. But when at sea, cigarettes were very cheap, time sometimes hung heavy so daily consumption was increased to 60. At sea the total daily number remained 60, but on return home he had no difficulty reducing the number to 20. In the summertime he was sometimes able to eliminate smoking altogether. Then he sought our help to rid himself of the habit entirely because of chronic bronchitis and also because the variations in his smoking pattern confused him.

In this case too, environment directed the smoking pattern. He was healthy enough to smoke 60 cigarettes a day at sea and could afford it. The pleasure of smoking seemed subordinate to other factors such as the pleasure of earning money by reducing the number of cigarettes while at home.

Example 3 We found exactly the same pattern in a 25-year-old volunteer in Korea. This patient smoked 60 cigarettes daily when in Korea where cigarettes were so inexpensive. In Sweden he limited himself to 20. In both places his smoking gave him full satisfaction.

We have had many patients at the clinics who varied the number of cigarettes smoked according to their environment. For example, they smoked 40 cigarettes daily when at work but only a few during their vacation or refrained entirely when doing manual outdoor work.

How can boys and girls be expected to reject cigarette smoking when they are constantly exposed to cigarette advertising and see smoking by parents, teachers, group leaders, actors and actresses on the stage, in movies, and on television, and by public figures, and even by religious leaders?

How can our young men and women who serve in the armed forces fail to accept cigarette smoking as "the thing to do" when cigarettes are available to them on every hand and when troops in training or on maneuvers are given not a rest but a cigarette break with the suggestion that they "light up"? If they are not regular smokers when they enter service, they almost certainly will be when they come out.

SOME PROGRESS BEING MADE

In spite of all this some progress is being made. Some magazines and newspapers and a few radio and television stations no longer accept cigarette advertising. The airlines have stopped the distribution of cigarettes with meals. Armed service hospitals in the United States have discontinued the distribution of cigarettes to patients. After colleges began to protest the advertising of cigarettes in campus publications and the sponsorship by cigarette companies of the broadcasting of intercollegiate sports, the tobacco companies discontinued this type of advertising. This seemed a commendable recognition of public responsibility until a spokesman for the industry said that it was done because cigarette smoking is for adults, not for children.

The American Medical Association has taken a positive position concerning the serious health hazard of cigarette smoking and recommends that programs be developed to disseminate vital health education material on the hazards of smoking to all age groups through all available means of communication. Many state medical societies are urging individual physicians, hospitals, and other medical institutions and organizations to take a leadership role in discouraging cigarette smoking. The Council of the California Medical Association has recommended not only that physicians should instruct and advise patients not to smoke but also that the physicians themselves should set an example of abstention. The Minnesota State Medical Society has requested all hospitals to prohibit smoking except in areas specifically designated for that purpose. The American Academy of Pediatrics passed a similar resolution. The American College of Physicians, which includes in its membership approximately 15,000 specialists in internal medicine, at its annual meeting in 1968 passed the following resolution:

> The Board of Regents not only strongly supports the warnings on the danger of the use of tobacco issued by the Surgeon General of the Public Health Service but, in addition, urges all members of the American College of Physicians to participate in educational efforts that will reduce the use of tobacco and, further, that the American College of Physicians recommend to the tobacco industry and to the Congress that cigarette advertising be banned on television.

Newspapers, magazines, and the news services of radio and television, in spite of substantial income from cigarette advertising, report accurately and fully on significant scientific work concerning the hazards of smoking. And one major commercial network, as well as the National Educational Television network, has produced several hour-long programs on this subject. Increasingly major newspapers as well are speaking out frankly and forcefully on this subject.

Schools are rapidly adding to their instructional programs significant information concerning the effects of tobacco upon health. This is tremendously important because teachers who are able to influence children not to smoke can do more to prevent illness, disability, and premature death from cancer, heart disease, bronchitis, and emphysema than the most skilled physicians can do by the treatment of patients who develop these diseases. In some schools and colleges student groups are concerning themselves with this problem. Most youth-serving organizations are cooperating in this effort.

Business organizations are beginning to consider the effects of smoking upon the efficiency of their employees. We have noted (page 130) the report that "Top Executives Heed Warnings to Stop Smoking." Reports of other efforts to reduce smoking in business organizations include the following:

At the World Conference on Smoking and Health, the chairman of the board of directors of the Franklin National Bank of New York rose to say:

> I would like to discuss for a few moments the most important area that has been covered by the reports that I have heard here this afternoon. That area has to do with business cooperation. I urge business corporations to consider a ban on smoking by their employees during business hours as part of their corporate responsibility in running efficient and profitable enterprises for their shareholders.
>
> Our bank, the Franklin National Bank, with seventy-eight branches in this Metropolitan area, four years ago next month placed a ban on smoking by our officers, our employees and our directors. This ban has been in effect without violation during that entire period.
>
> To our directors I said, "You have to set the example: you cannot smoke at any committee meetings, at any director's meetings, at any bank business meetings." They all agreed.
>
> I went next to the senior officers and told them the same thing. Then I did what was one of the most difficult things

that I ever had to do; that was to tell all of the other officers in the bank, who now number some four or five hundred, that this ban was going to be in effect.

On two previous occasions, seven years ago and a dozen years ago, I tried this on more or less of a voluntary basis. We had ashtrays removed. I spoke to the staff about the hazards of smoking and the illnesses that could shorten their lives. But most of them very soon returned to their old habits. So when I spoke with them four years ago, I didn't try to frighten them. I said, "I'm not going to tell you that you are going to live five years less than you might. I'm not going to tell you about your illnesses. I'm not going to tell you about the suffering you and your families are going to encounter. I'm not going to tell you these things. But as Chief Executive Officer of this bank, my job is to see that it is run as profitably as possible, and my calculations indicate that we can increase our profits by one and one-half percent if we eliminate smoking. So from this moment smoking is eliminated."

This briefly is our story. I think that it is a serious responsibility on the part of all corporate management to see to it that their companies are run as profitably as possible, and I feel certain that they can increase their profits up to three percent by the elimination of smoking. In my opinion corporate management is negligent if they do not do something about this serious matter.

A different strategy to reduce smoking was reported in January, 1968, by the chairman of the board of the City Federal Savings and Loan Bank in Birmingham, Alabama. He offered a $10-a-month salary bonus to employees who did not smoke. Of 50 employees, 15 were nonsmokers, 29 decided to quit, 6 said they couldn't quit. At the end of two months 27 of the 29 had stopped smoking—2 had slipped back. "All the remaining smokers were women. Not a single man on the staff smoked; not a member of the bank's board does either."

Concerning the program the Chairman of the Board said,

> The $10 per non-smoker per month is a real investment. Look at these statistics: Women who smoked used to go to the lounge four or five times a day and would spend 10 minutes each visit.—They don't do it any more. It is time gained for the company. Furthermore, the risk of fire has been greatly reduced; the chance of a cigarette falling off an ashtray and burning a hole in a couch or in the carpet has been all but erased.
>
> Furthermore, people who don't smoke increase their life span by four or five years. That means we won't lose these employees and have to spend money training replacements. Bonuses to non-smokers this banker feels are good business.

At its meeting in December, 1968, the American Medical Association expanded its previous statement concerning the harmful effects of cigarette smoking by urging its members to "play a major role against cigarette smoking by personal example and by advice regarding the health hazards of smoking," and by directing the Association to "discourage smoking by means of public pronouncements and educational programs," and to "take a strong stand against smoking by every means at [its] command."

Fortunately, as the above examples indicate, physicians, teachers, and other informed and responsible individuals and groups are beginning to assume leadership roles in this problem. Leadership by American medicine and by health, educational, and youth-serving organizations cannot fail to influence individual behavior and group action. It took more than half a century, billions of dollars in cigarette advertising, and the encouragement of smoking in two world wars to make cigarette smoking popular. It will take time, determination, and coordinated effort to change this. As Mark Twain said, "A habit cannot be tossed out of the window; it must be coaxed down the stairs a step at a time." Eventually, the public interest and welfare will prevail.

COUNTERATTACKS

Why, in view of all the evidence of the harmful effects of cigarette smoking, do broadcasters, newspapers, and the public still refer to this as a controversy? The answer is, because the tobacco industry has planned it that way.

Tobacco companies have always been highly individualistic and competitive. They still are, but reports of harmful effects from smoking have modified this. An old, well-established, profitable, and respected industry was deeply concerned. As I commented some years ago: [1] "There is something definitely sad when an industry finds that what it has been doing is useless, or worse than useless—definitely harmful." This is particularly true of those who became engaged in the manufacture and promotion of cigarettes before the risks of smoking were known.

[1] New York Times Book Review, Nov. 24, 1963.

THE TIRC

With the indictment of cigarettes as a health hazard the industry was faced with a new problem: a threat to the business of all companies—a threat that called for industry-wide as well as individual company action. To plan a defense of their business, industry leaders sought the advice of distinguished public relations counsel. Their recommendation was that the industry employ a competent public relations firm to concentrate upon this problem: questioning the evidence and keeping the subject controversial. Pursuant to this advice a New York public relations firm has for more than a decade effectively carried out this mission. Another move of the industry, also on the advice of public relations counsel, was the establishment in 1953 of a research organization called the Tobacco Industry Research Committee (TIRC), recently rechristened the Tobacco Research Council. Clarence Cook Little, Sc.D., was employed as chairman of its Scientific Advisory Board and became the chief scientific spokesman for the industry. In this role Dr. Little has been most effective: questioning evidence and insisting that nothing has been proved and that more research is needed.[2]

The TIRC's Scientific Advisory Board, which has included in its membership some well-known and respected medical scientists, passes upon requests for grants from a research fund provided by the industry. This Advisory Board has no public relations function, but it provides a background of scientific authority for the statements made by its chairman. Former U.S. Senator Maurine Neuberger wrote that "the creation of the TIRC, 'the brainchild' of the tobacco industry's resourceful public-relations firm was a stroke of ingenuity. The TIRC furnished a mechanism by which millions of dollars could be spread among research institutions to purchase

[2] See Dr. Little's statement of 1944 regarding cigarette smoking, p. 21.

(albeit subtly and indirectly) good will for the tobacco industry throughout the scientific community." In addition to supporting its own research program, the tobacco industry in 1963 made a grant of $10 million—$2 million a year for five years—to the American Medical Association's Research Foundation. This grant was renewed in 1968 for an additional four years.

THE TOBACCO INSTITUTE

In 1958 the major tobacco companies inaugurated another joint effort: the Tobacco Institute. The purpose of this institute is "to promote better public understanding of the tobacco industry and its place in the national economy and to compile and disseminate information relating to the industry and the use of tobacco products." The institute is a trade association which serves as the public relations agent of the industry as a whole.

On the health question the Tobacco Institute's consistent theme is: "There has been no scientific proof that cigarette smoking causes human disease." On matters of federal legislation or regulation it serves as a most effective spokesman for the industry. As its president it had George V. Allen, head of the U.S. Information Agency under President Eisenhower, and it now has Earle C. Clements, former governor of Kentucky (1945–1948) and United States Senator (1950–1957). Senator Clements, a long-time personal friend of President Johnson, served as Senate Democratic Whip when Lyndon Johnson was Senate Majority Leader. Another leading spokesman on Capitol Hill for the tobacco industry's position has been U.S. Senator Thruston Morton of Kentucky, former Chairman of the Republican National Committee. Men of their prestige and influence are able to intercede most effectively with members of Congress and with government agencies. Under such leadership the influence of the tobacco industry with the federal government is tremendous.

It was thought that after the Surgeon General's Advisory Committee—all of whose members had been approved for appointment by the Tobacco Institute—had completed its work and released its Report on Smoking and Health, the position of the industry would be changed. But this has not happened. In fact, after a period of silence and "study," the tobacco industry began to attack the validity of the report and to try to undermine confidence in its conclusions. This effort was even carried to the floor of Congress in hearings on the cigarette-labeling bills. In spite of increasing evidence that not only supports but goes far beyond the original conclusions of the Surgeon General's Advisory Committee, these attacks have continued, and are in fact being intensified.

The Public Health Service's 1967 report to Congress, "The Health Consequences of Smoking," was characterized by the Tobacco Institute as "an inaccurate and misleading interpretation" of scientific findings. The institute added that "Numerous studies indicate that there is a constitutional predisposition to disease and that smoking may be merely a reflection of a type of person who may be susceptible to certain ills." [3]

Such attacks have no demonstrable influence upon medical or scientific opinion, but they help to keep the public confused and uncertain. Particularly effective for this purpose are certain statements from the *Congressional Record* that are widely and repeatedly publicized in news releases, articles, and books. That these statements may have been made by individuals testifying for the tobacco industry is rarely suspected.

The tobacco industry, with the leadership of the Tobacco Institute and the cooperation of individual tobacco companies, exerts tremendous influence upon government, communications media, and many business institutions and organizations. The effect on public opinion is vastly more far-reaching and influential than one would suspect.

[3] *New York Times*, Aug. 22, 1967.

INFLUENCE UPON GOVERNMENT

In Chapter 13 we noted how the Federal Trade Commission's proposed regulation to require a clear warning on cigarette packages and in cigarette advertising was blocked and Congress was prevailed upon to substitute a weak, inconspicuous warning label on cigarette packages and to prohibit any warning in cigarette advertising. One of the arguments against a warning in cigarette advertising was that it would be an infringement upon free enterprise and freedom of speech and that, if approved, it would be the beginning of government censorship of all advertising. The answer of the Federal Trade Commission was that this was a special situation in which the product advertised had been declared by the Public Health Service to be a serious health hazard when used as advertised. In spite of this, Congress enacted legislation acceptable to the tobacco industry instead of the legislation supported by the Public Health Service, the Federal Trade Commission, and the medical and health organizations that testified.

Tobacco state congressmen also succeeded in preventing for a year an appropriation recommended by the President's office for the support of a Public Health Service program to inform the public of the health hazards of smoking.

Pending in court at the time of this writing is the suit brought jointly by the tobacco industry and the broadcasting industry to reverse the Federal Communications Commission ruling that television and radio stations which carry cigarette advertising must provide a significant amount of time for messages concerning the health hazards of smoking.

Tobacco industry influence was partially successful also in its effort to prevent the display of anti-smoking posters on United States mail trucks during the month of February, 1968. These posters,

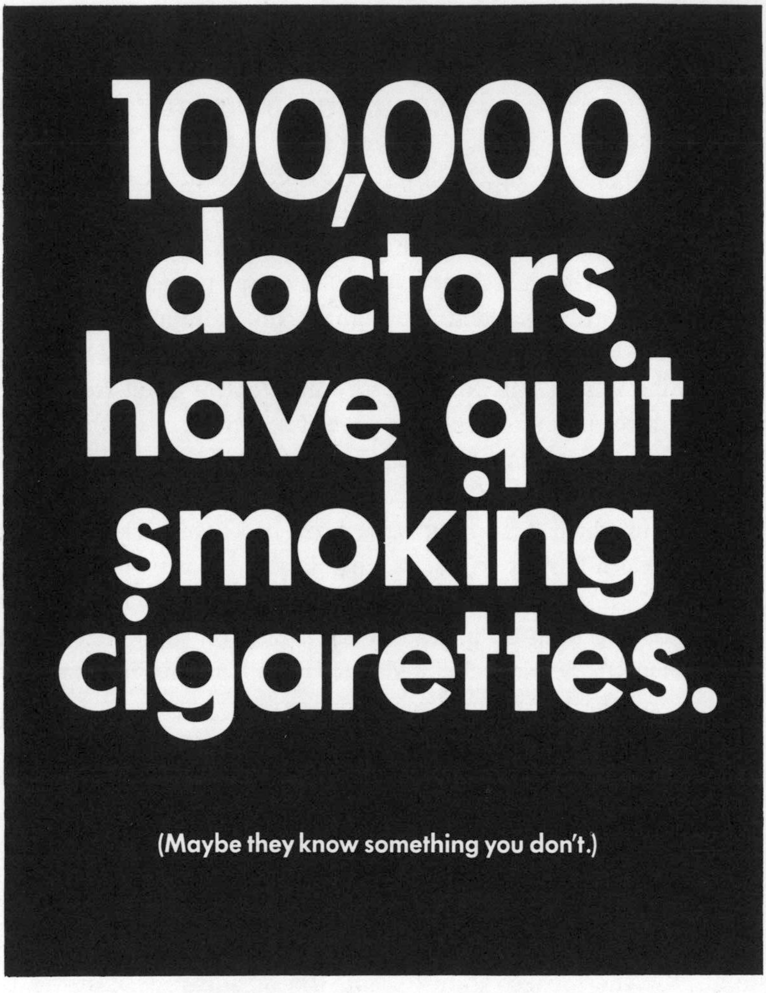

100,000 doctors have quit smoking cigarettes.

(Maybe they know something you don't.)

Figure 15.1. *A thought-provoking message concerning smoking. (Courtesy U.S. Department of Health, Education, and Welfare; Public Health Service.)*

which were prepared by the Public Health Service and approved by Post Office officials, stated: "100,000 Doctors Have Quit Smoking Cigarettes. (Maybe they know something you don't.)" An influential senator from a tobacco state sent telegrams to the

President, the Secretary of Health, Education, and Welfare, and the Postmaster General protesting the use of these posters and stating: "It is not the function of the Federal government to brainwash the American people in respect to their personal habits or anything else. I request you to immediately rescind your order dealing with these scare tactics." [4] The tobacco industry insisted that the statement that 100,000 doctors have stopped smoking is inaccurate because it is only an estimate and that the posters should so state (as though anyone would think that an actual count had been made and that exactly 100,000 doctors had stopped smoking). Yet the Public Health Service acceded to this demand. After other delays and a conference between the Secretary of Health, Education, and Welfare and the Postmaster General, the use of the posters was authorized. These tactics, however, reduced the time during which these posters were displayed from a month to less than two weeks.

State and local legislative and regulatory bodies are also under constant surveillance by lobbyists for the various groups that profit from the manufacture, promotion, and sale of tobacco products. For example, in the spring of 1965, prior to the passage of the Cigarette Labeling and Advertising Act, the Utah state legislature was considering a bill to require a warning in cigarette advertising. Since the Mormon church is opposed to smoking, the bill had strong support and seemed likely to pass. However, after the Utah Broadcasters' Association protested, the bill was tabled in committee.

INFLUENCE UPON NEWS MEDIA

All major commercial radio and television stations and networks and nearly all newspapers and magazines carry cigarette advertising. This advertising, upon which the tobacco industry is re-

---

[4] UPI release from Washington, Long Beach, Calif., Independent, Feb. 1, 1968.

ported to spend $300 million a year, constitutes an important source of revenue for these news media. It is natural therefore that they would want to conform to the wishes of the tobacco industry. In fact, it is surprising that they report evidence concerning the hazards of cigarette smoking as frankly and as fully as they do. Of course, in deference to the cigarette industry, they usually also publish derogatory comments from the Tobacco Institute on the scientific work reported.

INFLUENCE UPON OTHER BUSINESS INSTITUTIONS AND ORGANIZATIONS

The $8 billion tobacco industry has dealings with and influence upon many other businesses and institutions in our society. Banks and other financial institutions frequently have large investments in tobacco company stocks and bonds. The same is true of insurance companies, some of which sell insurance to tobacco companies and their employees. The health education materials of such companies may make little or no mention of the health hazards of smoking.

At the New York World's Fair the American Cancer Society proposed to include in its exhibit in the Hall of Science information about cigarette smoking and cancer. This exhibit was not accepted. The reason given was that it was not scientific. An unofficial explanation, however, was that a commission concerned with the Fair included in its membership the president of a tobacco company and that he might be offended by such an exhibit.

Throughout the country buses, subway cars, and railroad trains carry numerous cigarette advertisements, but rarely, if ever, among their "public service messages" does one see anything about the hazards of cigarette smoking. In the past, requests by the American Cancer Society for permission to place cards telling about the hazards of smoking in New York subway cars were always refused. Some years ago, however, subway cars carried cards stating that the House of Delegates of the American Medical Association has never said that cigarette smoking is harmful. At the time this statement was true, *but* its implication was misleading because up to that date the American Medical Association had never considered the smoking question. When it did so, several years later, the House of Delegates voted, without any recorded negative votes, that "cigarette smoking is a serious health hazard."

A suggestion that this attitude may be changing is the recent approval of a request from the New York City Health Department —with strong support by a member of the City Council—to place cards about the hazards of cigarette smoking in New York City subway cars and buses.

After the Federal Trade Commission began to report on the tar and nicotine in cigarettes, tobacco companies are reported to have appealed to the retail food and drugs industries not to display "at point of purchase" the FTC's "relative tar and nicotine ratings of cigarette brands."

INFLUENCE UPON PUBLIC THINKING

A number of competent public relations firms are employed by the tobacco industry to influence public thinking relative to the health hazards of smoking. Some of the methods used are:

News releases   News releases give nationwide publicity to medical articles which seem to question the relation of smoking to lung cancer, coronary disease, emphysema, or other diseases, or which suggest other possible causes of these diseases. The extent to which such propaganda carries is illustrated by the remark of the driver of the one and only taxi in a small town in northern Minnesota near which we have a summer cabin. His remark was that he had heard that "a German doctor said that cigarette smoking does not cause lung cancer." That was to him a welcome message because it eased his mind about continuing his heavy smoking. The German medical journal in which this report was published later repudiated the article, but he, of course, never heard of that.

Special articles   Special articles cast doubt upon the reliability of the studies and reports that conclude that cigarette smoking is harmful. Recent examples of such articles have appeared in *Barron's National Business and Financial Weekly*, in *Marketing Communications*, in *True* magazine and in the *National Enquirer*. The *Barron's* article was an editorial in the October 2, 1967, issue attacking the evidence that cigarette smoking is harmful and questioning the actions of the Public Health Service, the Federal Trade Commission, and the Federal Communications Commission. It referred to those who are working on this health problem as "witch doctors." This article was reprinted as a full-page advertisement by the Tobacco Institute in major newspapers throughout the country.

The *True* magazine article in January, 1968, is a restatement of the arguments regularly used to throw doubt on the conclusion that cigarette smoking causes lung cancer. The article is based primarily upon statements of tobacco industry witnesses at the hearings on the cigarette-labeling bills. It concludes: "There is absolutely no proof that smoking causes human cancer." This article was reprinted and widely distributed with the statement: "As a leader in your profession and community, you will be interested in reading this story from the January issue of *True* magazine about one of today's most controversial issues—The Editors." The article in *Marketing Communications*, November, 1967, has as a major title "Winstons Surge Up Front"—and a subtitle "The Health Scare? Forget It."

The article in the *National Enquirer*, New York, March 3, 1968, carries the following heading on its front page: [5]

Most Medical Experts Say:
· CIGARET CANCER LINK IS BUNK
—70,000,000 Smokers Falsely Alarmed

Books Books expand on the theme of the above articles. Two such books appeared in 1966, one by an American, Lloyd Mallan: *It Is Safe to Smoke*,[6] the other by an Englishman, C. Harcourt Kitchin: *You May Smoke*.[7] The Mallan book was highly publicized and promoted. Both books raise the usual questions concerning the evidence about the effects of smoking. In addition, the Mallan book contains extensive excerpts from the *Congressional Record* of testimony given by tobacco industry witnesses at the hearings on the cigarette-labeling bills. In a press interview reported by the *Washington Post*, Mr. Mallan said he did "not particularly like the title and had 'protested at first' to his publisher." He said: "My intention is not to encourage people who have stopped smoking to start again. Certainly I would not want young people to start smoking if they have not already done so." [8]

The *New York Times* review of the book said: "What the book finally comes to is that certain kinds of filter cigarettes are less harmful than others.—What he's given us is a puff for the industry." [9] The publishers discontinued sales of this book after the Deceptive Practices Division of the Federal Trade Commission began investigating the advertising.[10]

I mention these articles and books not because of their importance but as illustrations of the type of propaganda that is appearing

---

[5] For an explanation of the sponsorship of these articles and an analysis of their content, see Appendix C.

[6] Lloyd Mallan, "It Is Safe to Smoke," Hawthorn Books, New York, 1966.

[7] C. Harcourt Kitchin, "You May Smoke," Award Books, New York, 1966.

[8] The Washington Post, Mar. 1, 1967.

[9] New York Times Book Review, Jan. 22, 1967.

[10] The Wall Street Journal, Mar. 26, 1968.

MAIL   THIS   **VIETNAM**
ORDER BLANK TO: **ORDER BLANK**

The American Tobacco Co., 245 Park Avenue, New York, N.Y. 10017
          Enclose check or money order in proper amount payable to
The American Tobacco Company. Shipment of tax-free cigarettes will be
made to Vietnam (or other areas of the Far East—Thailand, Korea, Laos,
Burma, etc.) through the Army or Fleet Post Office (APO or FPO) by AIR,
Space Available Mail.
          Your name and address will be printed on a label which will be
inserted under the cellophane of each package indicating shipment is a
gift from you. Acknowledgment card from recipient addressed to you will
also be placed in each carton.

SHIP TO _____
(Please Print)   Military unit or individual (name, rank, serial no.)

ADDRESS _____

YOUR NAME _____

ADDRESS _____

CITY   STATE   ZIP CODE

Quantity	Brand	Delivered Price
_____ (50 pkgs.)	LUCKY STRIKE — Regular	$5.53
_____ (50 pkgs.)	LUCKY FILTERS — King Size	5.73
_____ (50 pkgs.)	LUCKY STRIKE Menthol — King Size	5.73
_____ (50 pkgs.)	LUCKY FILTERS — 100's	6.22
_____ (50 pkgs.)	LUCKY STRIKE Menthol — 100's	6.22
_____ (50 pkgs.)	PALL MALL — King Size	5.73
_____ (50 pkgs.)	PALL MALL Filter Tipped — 100's	6.22
_____ (50 pkgs.)	PALL MALL Menthol — 100's	6.22
_____ (50 pkgs.)	TAREYTON — King Size	5.73
_____ (50 pkgs.)	TAREYTON — 100's	6.22
_____ (50 pkgs.)	CARLTON	5.73
_____ (50 pkgs.)	MONTCLAIR	5.73
_____ (50 pkgs.)	HALF and HALF	5.73
_____ (50 pkgs.)	BULL DURHAM	5.73

ALL PRICES ARE SUBJECT TO CHANGE WITHOUT NOTICE

with increasing frequency. It is important that the public recognize such publications for what they are and discriminate between responsible reporting and propaganda for profit.

Cigarettes for our soldiers   Cigarette manufacturers offering to send tax-free shipments to military personnel in the Far East would seem to be performing a patriotic service. They are, in fact, promoting the smoking habit among the nation's fittest young men and women.

The accompanying figure illustrates a sample, hard-to-resist "Vietnam order blank." The background of this form was detailed in the April, 1967 issue of *Tobacco Reporter*, which stated that a ruling by the U.S. Treasury Department had made it possible for tobacco companies to send cigarettes overseas untaxed. Since then, virtually every cigarette manufacturer has initiated a program making it possible to ship gift "smokes" overseas at a cost of only 9 to 11 cents a pack.

A PERSONAL DECISION

The decision to smoke or not to smoke is one that each individual must make for himself. It is not proposed that the production or sale of cigarettes be prohibited. Cigarettes will continue to be available. The question is, How can those who are faced with this decision make a free and intelligent choice?

One must first of all understand the extent and the seriousness of the hazard. It is not enough to be vaguely informed; one must be *convinced* as doctors are convinced. Most people have heard of the risk of smoking but really know very little about it. If the "average smoker" could see, as doctors do, the hospital rooms, wards, and even buildings (particularly in Veterans Hospitals) filled with patients suffering from emphysema, heart disease, lung cancer, and other diseases attributable to smoking, he could not fail to be impressed with the tragic results of this habit. One can never really visualize the situation by reading, hearing, or even seeing pictures of it. Few people can work with or see such patients. The evidence must be studied, and sound and responsible medical advice on the subject heeded.

To make free and informed decisions it is essential that the encouragements and pressures to influence people to smoke be eliminated or at least drastically reduced. These pressures come from the desire to conform, from the social acceptance of smoking, from advertising, and from other subtle and frequently unrecognized "persuaders."

The desire to conform is innate in most people. One does not like to be different from the group of which he is a part. Many boys and girls start and continue to smoke because their associates smoke. A cigarette is offered. A refusal or hesitancy brings forth the question: "Aren't you one of us"; "Are you a baby"; or "Are you chicken"—"Come on, get with it." Even hippies, who pride themselves on being social nonconformists, are characterized by their group conformity in long, uncombed hair, in exotic, sloppy dress, in the use of drugs, and in the smoking of cigarettes and marijuana. To resist these pressures to smoke requires courage to be different and determination to be one's self. Models whom one admires and wishes to emulate, be these parents, older brothers or sisters, teachers, group leaders, or friends who do not smoke, set an important example. As Dr. Karl Evang, the Director General of Health Services of Norway, said at the World Conference on Smoking and Health, "One example is better than a thousand words, even if they are true."

The social acceptability and the prevalence of smoking are constant encouragements to smoke. It took years of commercial promotion to develop this situation, and it is difficult to change. However, cigarettes are provided less frequently at social events, and an increasing number of educational, recreational, religious, and youth-serving organizations are discouraging smoking. Also business organizations, as they recognize the increased amount of illness, disability, and loss of time due to smoking, are beginning to discourage smoking among their employees.

CIGARETTE ADVERTISING

Advertising has been tremendously effective in promoting cigarette smoking. One can hardly look at television, magazines, and newspapers or listen to radio without being exposed to attractive, appealing advertisements for this or that brand of cigarettes. Concerning this advertising, the Federal Trade Commission said in its report to Congress in the summer of 1967:

> Cigarette advertising reaches virtually all Americans who can either read, or understand the spoken word. Cigarettes are advertised on both network and spot television, on radio, in magazines and newspapers, in outdoor media, and by means of many types of point of sale advertising aids. So pervasive is cigarette advertising that it is virtually impossible for Americans of almost any age to avoid it. For example, the morning radio news broadcasts are often preceded or followed by spot announcement for a cigarette brand. Outdoor billboards, trains, and buses carry advertising visible to both children and adults on their way to work or school. Restaurants and drugstores often have advertising decals for cigarettes on entrance doors and a variety of other display material, such as wall clocks and change counter mats. Many of the daytime and evening television programs are sponsored by cigarette manufacturers; and numerous magazines and newspapers read by the whole family contain cigarette advertising.

The Federal Trade Commission reported also that during the week of January 11, 1967, 60 network television programs sponsored in whole or in part by cigarette manufacturers played before audiences that included 151 million viewers aged 2 to 12 and 141 million viewers aged 13 to 17. (A viewer in this context is one person watching one show. If one person watches five shows, he would be counted as five viewers.) The Commission report concluded: "The cigarette advertisements, especially on television and radio, have been successful in their subtle but effective attempts to persuade teenagers to smoke despite the known health hazards."

At the World Conference on Smoking and Health, Senator Robert F. Kennedy said: "Nearly $300 million a year is spent in the United States alone on television, radio and newspaper efforts to start young people smoking and continue others in the habit. We cannot seriously expect to make major inroads in people's smoking habits while $300 million a year is being spent to increase the numbers of those addicted. Action is needed to limit and counteract this massive onslaught." The following day Senator Kennedy introduced two bills into Congress relating to advertising. One was to strengthen the warning on cigarette packages to state "Warning: Cigarette Smoking Is Dangerous to Health and May Cause Death from Cancer and Other Diseases," and to require that this warning appear also in cigarette advertising. The other bill would authorize the Federal Communications Commission to regulate the time and type of program on which cigarette advertising may appear, and to control the overall volume of cigarette advertising as well. In presenting these bills Senator Kennedy said, "Something must be done now to control the advertising which encourages young people to start smoking at the rate of 1,500,000 a year. In my judgment industry self-regulation of advertising has been totally inadequate. Therefore, I am introducing these two bills relating to cigarette advertising."

In a similar vein Mr. Emerson Foote, former president of the largest advertising firm in this country, said: "Basically, the promotion of cigarette smoking is a clear application of the principle of the primacy of profits over people. In one way or another the disasterous effects of cigarette advertising on the health of our people, present and future, must be done away with."

On this subject the Board of Directors of the American Cancer Society in October, 1967, adopted the following resolution:

> Advertising is too persuasive, too valid and vital a part of our American life, to be used in the sale of such a lethal product as the cigarette. In full awareness of the seriousness of this problem, some influential publishers and some broadcasters have already voluntarily banned cigarette advertising.
>
> Therefore, we, the Board of Directors of the American Cancer Society, Inc., recommend that all cigarette advertising in all media be terminated. It is hoped that this goal will be achieved by voluntary self-regulation and that governmental action will not be necessary.
>
> Cigarette smoking is not the result of an advertising conspiracy. It is an extremely complex problem involving many little understood behavioral and pharmacological factors. But the elimination of cigarette advertising may do much to destroy the social acceptability of this dangerous habit. It will make giving up smoking easier for many, and it will stop the constant media pressures on the young to start smoking.
>
> The end of cigarette advertising will not be accomplished immediately. Many important actions which counterbalance advertising must be supported until the final goal is achieved.
>
> Cigarette smoking must remain a matter of individual choice but we want the choice to be not only informed, but free from seductive advertising appeals.

In March, 1968, the American College of Physicians recommended "to the tobacco industry and to the Congress that cigarette advertising be banned on television." Until this is done, each one can do much to protect himself by analyzing and considering the purpose of the advertising to which we are all exposed.

Other persuaders, some subtle and some not so subtle, include the use of cigarettes as "props" on the stage, on television, and in advertisements of products other than cigarettes. Smoking in such situations may well have a greater subconscious influence upon smoking attitudes and practices than overt advertising. The ubiquitous ashtrays and matches are also persuaders. Then there are the sample packages of cigarettes distributed at banquets, conventions, and even on street corners by attractive young women. The coupons in some cigarette packages encourage the purchase of more. Such coupons were extensively utilized in Britain when cigarette advertising was banned on radio and television.

THE COST OF SMOKING

Another consideration that should be realistically faced in making a decision to smoke or not to smoke is the cost. If a man smokes a pack a day from the age of twenty to the age of sixty-five, the cost will be about $6,000. If he marries a girl who smokes a pack a day, the cost will be twice that amount, or about $12,000. If either one or both smokes more than a pack a day, the cost will be proportionately greater.

Vastly more serious, however, for most smokers than the cost of cigarettes are the illnesses, the disabilities, and the premature deaths that result from smoking. For those who smoke one to two packs a day, days lost from work by men are 48 percent more, and by women 79 percent more, than for nonsmokers; days spent in bed because of illness are 22 percent more for men and 57 percent more for women who smoke than for nonsmokers; days of restricted activity are 39 percent more for men and 48 percent more for women who smoke than for nonsmokers; hospitalization is 50 percent more for heavy smokers than for nonsmokers. (See Chapter 9.) The costs of medical care, drugs, and hospitalization for these excess illnesses are tremendous, for many catastrophic— particularly for those who develop chronic bronchitis and emphysema, heart disease, ulcers of the stomach or duodenum, cancer, or strokes.

In addition there is the loss of income during the long illness and the loss of life while one is still of employable age, i.e., under sixty-five.

If the men who die prematurely between twenty-five and sixty-five because of smoking had an average income of $10,000 per year, the loss to their families from early death attributable to smoking would be $18,000 for those who smoked less than a half a pack a day; $26,000 for those who smoked half a pack to a pack a day; $31,000 for those who smoked a pack to two packs a day; and $49,000 for those who smoked two or more packs a day. For those with incomes more or less than $10,000 a year, the loss would be proportionate.

TABLE 16.1 **Years of life lost between 25 and 65 (cigarette smokers in excess of nonsmokers)**

Cigarettes smoked per day	Years lost
1–9	1.8
10–19	2.6
20–39	3.1
40+	4.9

SOURCE: Computed from E. Cuyler Hammond, Report to World Conference on Smoking and Health, Sept. 11, 1967: ''World Costs of Cigarette Smoking in Disease, Disability, and Death.''

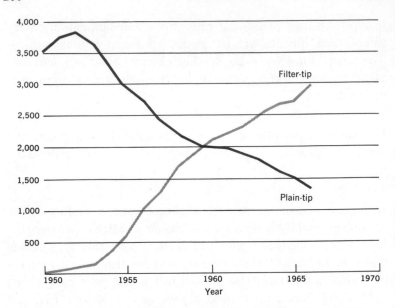

Figure 16.1. *Annual consumption of plain-tip and filter-tip cigarettes per person 18 years or over, United States, 1950–1966. (Source: U.S. Department of Agriculture.)*

Sir George Godber, the Chief Medical Officer of the British Ministry of Health, reported at the World Conference on Smoking and Health that in Great Britain there are 50,000 excess deaths a year attributable to cigarette smoking and that this represents an annual loss of 150,000 working years—that is, deaths before the age of sixty-five. This is an average of three working years lost for each smoker who died. As shown in Table 16.1, this is the average loss of working years in this country by men who smoke between one and two packs a day and die before sixty-five.

Since there are an estimated 300,000 deaths annually in the United States attributable to cigarette smoking—six times as many as in Great Britain—the corresponding annual working years lost (i.e., an average of three years per person) would be 900,000. If the average earned income of those who die prematurely as a result of cigarette smoking—most of whom are men—is $8,000, the annual loss to the economy would be $7.2 billion, or almost as much as the total annual revenue from tobacco and tobacco products. If the average income of those who die is $5,000, the total loss to the economy would be $4.5 billion. And these figures do not include the loss of income from disability or the costs of medical care and hospitalization, or the $80 million property damage from fires—to say nothing of forest fires—caused by cigarette smoking or by matches used in cigarette smoking.[1]

LESS HARMFUL CIGARETTES

The demand for filter-tip cigarettes is clear evidence that most smokers are anxious to reduce the hazard of their smoking. In 1952 filter-tip cigarettes made up only 1 percent of sales; fifteen years later they accounted for 70 percent of cigarette sales. The increase is doubtless because the public believes that filters provide at least some protection against the harmful substances in the smoke. For some filters this is true, for others untrue.

The amounts of harmful substances in tobacco smoke—tars, nicotine, and certain gases—are dependent primarily upon the type and the amount of tobacco used, the process of "curing," the addition of certain chemicals to the tobacco, the temperature of burning, the way it is smoked, and the effectiveness of filtration. By altering these factors, cigarette manufacturers can control most of the ingredients of the smoke.

Actually, considerable improvement in this regard was made about ten years ago.[2] Between 1957 and 1961, the tar content of all

[1] Estimate for 1965 by the National Fire Protection Association.
[2] See Reader's Digest articles by Lois Mattox Miller and James Monahan, July, 1957; August, 1957; November, 1959; July, 1961; August, 1963; and November, 1966.

major brands and the nicotine content of most major brands were reduced, and in most filter-tip cigarettes were reduced substantially. Since 1961 about half of comparable types of major brand cigarettes have shown further though small reductions; the others have shown small increases of tar and nicotine content.

During this period six new brands with low tar and low nicotine content have been marketed and several of these have become quite popular. Unfortunately, for many smokers the increased margin of safety provided by many filters has been more than offset by the introduction and intensive promotion of extra-long 100-millimeter cigarettes, some of which, in spite of filters, are very high in both tar and nicotine.

The tobacco industry contends that there is *no proof* that reducing the tar-nicotine content of cigarettes makes them less harmful. This is correct. However, since the harmful effects of smoking are directly related to dosage, there is every reason to think that this is true. Furthermore, fewer cancers develop in mice if their skins are painted with tars from low tar–low nicotine cigarettes than from high tar–high nicotine cigarettes. Also there is epidemiological evidence that men who smoke low tar–low nicotine cigarettes have less cough and expectoration than men who smoke other brands. Dr. George Moore, director of New York State's Roswell Park Memorial (Cancer) Institute says: "If the industry would use filters that would reduce the delivery of tar to a level of 15 milligrams per cigarette or below, such cigarettes would be approximately half as dangerous as the average cigarette."

It has been suggested that if smokers switch to low tar–low nicotine cigarettes they will smoke proportionately more in their desire for the same effects. Experience has shown that this does not happen and that those who do change generally smoke the same amount as previously. In fact, the switch to low tar–low nicotine cigarettes may be a first step toward quitting.

For cigarette smokers who are unwilling or unable to give up the habit, a switch to pipes, cigars, or low tar–low nicotine cigarettes is desirable. Individuals who wish to select low tar–low nicotine cigarettes should seek information from the U.S. Public Health Service, the Federal Trade Commission, or a local health department or health agency about the results of the most recent Federal Trade Commission tests of the cigarettes on the American market.

The importance of specific information instead of the selection of just any filter-tip cigarette is apparent from the tests that have been made (see Appendix D). For example, a smoker who switches from *nonfilter* cigarettes to certain *filter-tip* brands may get a dose of approximately 25 percent more tar and nicotine. On the other hand, if he switches from other *nonfilter* brands to certain *filter* brands—some even king-size—he will get 50 to 75 percent less tar and nicotine.

The addition of menthol to tobacco gives the smoke a medicated taste but does not affect the tar-nicotine content or in any way reduce the harmful effects of smoking.

Cigarette filters contain several materials, frequently cellulose acetate, to retain particulate material in the smoke which passes through it. In general, the effectiveness of a filter depends on how tightly it is packed. Thus, the effectiveness of filters is roughly proportional to their weight. This creates a problem because the more tightly a filter is packed, the more difficult it is to draw smoke through it. Smoking cigarettes with very tightly packed filters is said to be similar to smoking a lead pencil. Loosening up the filter will make puffing easier but will also let through more tar and nicotine. Some filters containing activated charcoal are reported to reduce the phenols in the smoke, thereby decreasing the toxic effect of the smoke upon the cilia.

Another fact that smokers should know is that tobacco itself is a good filter and that because of this the amount of tar and nicotine in the smoke from the last one-third of a cigarette is as great as that from the first two-thirds. The hazard of smoking, therefore, could be reduced by *half* if one smoked only half of each cigarette.

Why, with these possibilities of producing less harmful cigarettes, do tobacco companies not do so? And why do they object to giving the public information about the tar-nicotine content of the various brands of cigarettes? Certainly the tobacco companies do not wish to harm people. They do, however, wish to sell cigarettes. Since tar provides "flavor" in cigarette smoke, there is fear that if the tar content of a cigarette is too low, people may not smoke it. Also if the nicotine is too low, the cigarettes may not give the "kick" or satisfaction to which a regular smoker is accustomed. Furthermore, since the nicotine is believed to be the addictive constituent of the smoke, if the nicotine content is reduced it may be easier for the smoker to stop altogether.

Concerning less harmful cigarettes Dr. Ernest Wynder of the Sloan-Kettering Cancer Research Institute says: "Since a great many smokers will continue the habit in spite of all the evidence presented to them, it becomes a matter of urgency to make tobacco smoking less harmful. We hold it as a matter of sound realism that much practical progress can be made in the area of tobacco research." [3]

Much research is in progress by tobacco companies, government, and independent investigators to find a way to make cigarette smoking less harmful and still acceptable. Some progress has been made in this direction, but a cigarette that can be *demonstrated* to be "safe" and still acceptable to smokers is not in sight.

[3] Ernest L. Wynder and Dietrich Hoffman, "Tobacco and Tobacco Smoke," Academic Press, Inc., New York, 1967.

IF YOU MUST SMOKE

The best health advice you can give to those who do not smoke is "Never start the habit"; and to those who do smoke, "Stop completely." However, for those who are unable or unwilling to stop, the U.S. Public Health Service has prepared a pamphlet which says that by following a few simple rules, one can reduce the hazard:

1 Smoke cigarettes with less tar and nicotine.
2 Do not smoke cigarettes all the way down: the last third of a cigarette yields twice as much tar and nicotine as the first third.
3 Take fewer draws on each cigarette. The "extra puffs" in longer cigarettes are "extra perils" for you.
4 Reduce inhaling: do not consciously inhale.
5 Smoke fewer cigarettes each day. [Some suggestions to help with this are included in the aforementioned pamphlet.[4] (See also Appendix D, page 231.)]

MORE RESEARCH

The tobacco industry keeps insisting that more research is necessary. This is true. More research *is* needed—but *not* research to demonstrate the hazards of smoking; these have been clearly established. It is needed to further identify the specific substances in tobacco smoke that damage human health; to show how these affect the body; to improve the treatment of the diseases caused by smoking—now tragically ineffective; to determine why people take up smoking and continue to smoke; to develop less harmful ciga-

[4] "If You Must Smoke: Five Ways to Reduce the Risk of Smoking." Public Health Service Publication No. 1786, National Clearinghouse for Smoking and Health, Arlington, Va. 22203, August, 1968.

rettes; and finally, and optimally, to help smokers give up the habit entirely.

Research in all these areas must be encouraged and supported. This ongoing research, however, cannot be used as an excuse for continuing to smoke or as a reason for not acting on the basis of available information to reduce this health hazard.

A PERSONAL DECISION

The conclusion that cigarette smoking is a serious health hazard is inescapable. The scientific data, some of which are presented in this book, as well as the statements of responsible medical and health authorities in this country and abroad, leave no doubt about this. Yet cigarette smoking is widespread and socially acceptable and to many smokers it provides certain satisfactions. Most of these appear to be psychological rather than physiological, although the drug effect of nicotine is probably an important factor in the strongly addicted smoker.

Smoking also is big business, promoted by extensive, attractive, and persuasive advertising and by the ablest public relations that an $8 billion business can provide. And effective political lobbies guard against legislative actions or administrative controls that may interfere with this business.

The decision as to what to do about smoking is therefore up to the individual. As a behavioral phenomenon and a psychological habit it can be understood and changed. With adequate information and strong motivation—and in some cases with support and guidance—smoking can be avoided or controlled as one wishes. It is incumbent, however, on the individual to initiate his own self-directed, self-help program.

According to a report by the director of the National Clearing-house on Smoking and Health there were in 1968 1.5 million fewer cigarette smokers of all ages in the United States than in 1967. Even more impressive was the decrease in smoking among teen-agers. And perhaps of still greater importance is the fact that 45 percent of the teen-agers interviewed said that they *definitely* do not expect to begin smoking within the next five years, and another 34 percent said they *probably* will not do so.

This decline in smoking by teen-agers is encouraging not only because it will mean better health to those who have stopped and to those who have not started smoking but also because it indicates that the youth of this country are becoming informed and are beginning to think for themselves on this important health problem. Hopefully this represents the beginning of a trend that will not only continue among teen-agers but will have a salutary effect upon the smoking habits of adults.

If someone were able to develop a vaccine that would prevent 80 percent of lung cancers, would save an estimated 300,000 lives each year and would prevent a large amount of illness and disability, including 77 million lost work-days and 11 million cases of chronic illness each year, everybody would clamor for it.

Yet there is available to everyone not a vaccine but a simple procedure that not only will do all this but, in addition, will save one money and prevent a great deal of suffering. How can any rational person fail to utilize it?

The decision is yours.

SUGGESTED REFERENCES

1 *Smoking and Health,* Report of the Advisory Committee to the Surgeon General of the Public Health Service, U.S. Department of Health, Education, and Welfare, Washington, 1964.

The complete report of the Advisory Committee appointed by the Surgeon General to weigh all available evidence concerning the effects of smoking on health. An analysis of more than 4,000 reports. The most comprehensive and authoritative consideration of this important health problem ever made. A condensed summary is available free from local divisions and units of the American Cancer Society.

2 *The Health Consequences of Smoking: A Public Health Service Review: 1967,* and *Supplement 1968,* U.S. Department of Health, Education, and Welfare, Washington, 1967, 1968.

Reports to Congress in 1967 and 1968 of conclusions based upon research studies on this subject that have been published since the report on Smoking and Health by the Surgeon General's Advisory Committee in 1964.

3 *Smoking and Health:* Summary and Report of the Royal College of Physicians of London on Smoking in Relation to Cancer of the Lung and Other Diseases, Pitman Publishing Corporation, New York, 1962. (Available through the American Cancer Society.)

4 *The Canadian Smoking and Health Program,* 1967; and *Smoking and Health,* Reference Book, Canada, 1964, Department of National Health and Welfare, Ottawa, Canada.

5 *Task Force for Smoking and Health:* Report to the Surgeon General, U.S. Department of Health, Education, and Welfare, Washington, 1968. Reprinted by National Interagency Council on Smoking and Health, P.O. Box 3654, Central Station, Arlington, Virginia, 22203.

An analysis and report by a group of distinguished citizens concerning the smoking problem and what is being done about it, with recommendations as to what more can and should be done.

6 BEST, E. W. R., C. B. WALKER, P. M. BAKER, F. M. DELA-QUIS, J. T. McGREGOR AND A. C. McKENSIE: *Summary of a Canadian Study of Smoking and Health,* Canadian Department of Health and Welfare, Toronto, *Canadian Medical Association Journal,* vol. 96, p. 1104, Apr. 15, 1967.

Analysis of a six-year follow-up of Canadian veteran pension recipients to determine the relationship between residence, occupation, and smoking habits, and mortality from chronic diseases, particularly lung cancer.

7 HAMMOND, E. CUYLER: *Smoking in Relation to the Death Rates of One Million Men and Women*, Monograph 19, National Cancer Institute, Bethesda, Md., 1966.

   The most extensive and significant study of this subject ever made. Reprints may be obtained from the American Cancer Society.

8 *Cigarette Smoking and Health Characteristics*, National Center for Health Statistics, ser. 10, no. 34, U.S. Public Health Service, May, 1967.

   Statistics on the prevalence of selected chronic conditions, such as heart disease, bronchitis, emphysema, peptic ulcer; incidence of selected acute conditions, such as respiratory infectious, infective, and parasitic diseases; and days of disability by cigarette smoking habits, sex, and age.

9 NEUBERGER, MAURINE B.: *Smoke Screen—Tobacco and the Public Welfare*, Prentice-Hall, Inc., Englewood Cliffs, N.J., 1963.

   Excellent presentation by Senator Neuberger of the pertinent facts in cigarette promotion, advertising, government inaction, public and private inquiry, and research statistics on the relationship between tobacco and disease.

10 *Federal Trade Commission Report to Congress: Pursuant to the Federal Cigarette Labeling and Advertising Act.* Washington, 1968.

   A report concerning (1) the effectiveness of cigarette labeling, (2) practices and methods of cigarette advertising and promotion, and (3) recommendations for legislation which are deemed appropriate.

11 *The Development and Marketing of a Less Hazardous Cigarette*, Hearings before the Consumer Subcommittee of the

Committee on Commerce, U.S. Congress, 1967, U.S. Government Printing Office, Washington, 1968.

12 BLAKESLEE, ALTON L.: *It's Not Too Late to Stop Smoking*, Public Affairs Pamphlet, New York, 1966.

The reasons why it is worth the effort to stop smoking and ways of doing it.

13 READ, CLIFTON R.: *If You Want to Give Up Cigarettes*, American Cancer Society, 219 East 42nd Street, New York, N.Y. 10017, 1968.

An outline of suggestions (see Appendix D) that may be helpful to cigarette smokers who wish to stop. For more information contact the local office of the American Cancer Society.

14 SALBER, EVA J.: *Facts about Smoking and Health*, Science Research Associates, Inc., 259 East Erie Street, Chicago, 1964.

In this small book Dr. Salber not only distills some of the most significant aspects of her studies of smoking among high-school students in Newton, Mass., but also discusses evidence of the harmful effects of smoking, the reasons boys and girls smoke, and the changes that occurred in the smoking habits of a group of high-school students over a period of six months. The book concludes with suggestions as to how students can cooperate in programs to reduce smoking.

15 "National Forum on the Office Management of Smoking Problems: Diseases of the Chest," vol. 54, no. 3, September, 1968. American College of Chest Physicians, 112 East Chestnut Street, Chicago, Illinois.

A splendid, practical discussion by distinguished physicians experienced in aiding people who for medical or other reasons wish to give up smoking.

16 GOODMAN, HENRY A. (ed.): *World Conference on Smoking and Health: A Summary of the Proceedings.* Distributed by National Interagency Council on Smoking and Health, P.O. Box 3654, Central Station, Arlington, Va. 22203. Paperback: October, 1968.

A 300-page summary of the major papers and discussions at the World Conference on Smoking and Health, held in New York on September 11, 12, and 13, 1967—a conference attended by more than 500 delegates from 34 countries.

17 *Helping People to Stop Smoking Cigarettes,* American Cancer Society, 219 East 42nd Street, New York, N.Y. 10017, 1968.

Reports and comments, concerning experimental programs, that may be useful to communities wishing to establish their own programs.

18 *Your Teen-ager and Smoking,* American Medical Association, 535 No. Dearborn Street, Chicago, Ill.

19 LARSON, P. S., AND H. SILVETTE: *Experimental and Clinical Studies: Supplement I,* Williams and Wilkins Company, Baltimore, Md., 1968.

This book of 814 pages, a supplement to the original book of 932 pages published in 1961, is based upon some 6,000 articles on the subject of tobacco and its effect on health. The new volume gives special attention to clinical studies, and contains a complete index of cross references.

MATCHED PAIR ANALYSIS*

Deaths among 36,975 men who never smoked regularly, and 36,975 men currently smoking 20 or more cigarettes a day at enrollment in study.

TABLE B.1 **Deaths by age groups**

Age group	Never smoked regularly		Cigarettes 20+ a day	
	Number of men	Number of deaths	Number of men	Number of deaths
40–44	3,410	15	3,410	40
45–49	10,468	59	10,468	192
50–54	9,583	123	9,583	252
55–59	6,534	135	6,534	323
60–64	3,990	150	3,990	254
65–69	2,083	98	2,083	193
70–74	747	64	747	98
75–79	160	18	160	33
Total	36,975	662	36,975	1,385

* For an explanation of and reference to this study, see p. 32.

TABLE B.2 Deaths by causes (age range 40–79)

Underlying cause of death	Number of deaths	
	Never smoked regularly	Cigarettes 20+ a day
Cancer (total)	96	261
Lung	12	110
Buccal cavity; pharynx	1	3
Larynx	0	3
Esophagus	0	6
Bladder	1	2
Pancreas	6	16
Liver; biliary passages	1	7
Stomach	9	10
Colon; rectum	20	25
Other specified sites	43	64
Site unknown	3	15
Heart and circulatory (total)	401	854
Coronary	304	654
Other heart	30	64
Aortic aneurysm	8	30
Cerebral vascular	44	84
Other circulatory	15	22
Other diseases (total)	73	127
Emphysema	1	15
Gastric ulcer	3	5
Cirrhosis of liver	9	17
Other specified diseases	59	86
Ill-defined diseases	1	4
Accidents; violence; suicides	58	66
Total death certificates	628	1,308
No death certificates	34	77
Grand total	662	1,385

ATTACKS ON THE EVIDENCE ON SMOKING AND HEALTH

APPENDIX C

PRO-SMOKING ARTICLES AREN'T NECESSARILY ALL THAT THEY SEEM TO BE [1]

*Sen. Magnuson Asks Inquiry Into Story by PR Writer;
Tobacco Men Buy Reprints*

It seemed like a windfall for the tobacco industry. "To Smoke or Not to Smoke—That Is Still the Question" was the title of an article in the January issue of True magazine. There was little question which side of the issue the article took.

Dismissing statistical evidence of cancer hazards in smoking cited by the U.S. Surgeon General, the article concluded, "At the mo-

[1] Article from The Wall Street Journal, by Ronald Kessler, staff reporter, New York, Mar. 21, 1968.

ment, all we can say for sure is that the cause of cancer isn't known and that there is absolutely no proof that smoking causes human cancer."

The story was widely promoted in advertisements, and reprints were mailed to about 600,000 "opinion makers" around the nation. Not surprisingly, five of the six major tobacco companies mailed reprints to their employes and shareholders.

The article couldn't have presented the tobacco industry's case better if it had been written by the industry. And though there's no proof the industry did that, the circumstances surrounding its publication are interesting.

"Bunk" says a tabloid

The author, Stanley Frank, is an employe of Hill & Knowlton Inc., long-time public relations representative for the industry's Tobacco Institute Inc. The reprints and ads, ostensibly a True promotion, actually were paid for and handled by Tiderock Corp., a second public relations firm hired by the Tobacco Institute last October.

More recently, the March 3 issue of a sensational tabloid, the National Enquirer, carried a story under the headline "Cigaret Cancer Link is Bunk." The byline read "Charles Golden," but Nat Chrzan, editor of the Enquirer, says the author was Mr. Frank. "Charles Golden doesn't exist," Mr. Chrzan says. "It's all perfectly legal."

Mr. Frank at first flatly denied authorship of the Enquirer story; a week later he conceded that he had written it. "You've got me on that one," he said. As to the True article, Mr. Frank says he submitted it last April, while he was a free-lance writer, whereas he didn't join the public relations agency until October. True and Hill & Knowlton give a like account of the chronology, although the public relations director of a major tobacco company says he

understands that Mr. Frank was working on the True story last
fall.

Congressional sources say the tobacco industry is mounting an
aggressive new campaign to counter medical evidence that cigaret
smoking is damaging to health. The Surgeon General has been
asked by Sen. Warren G. Magnuson, chairman of the Senate
Commerce Committee, to investigate the True article and the
legality of the reprints.

Dispute over a book

A similar dispute arose early last year on publication of the book It
Is Safe To Smoke by Hawthorn Books Inc., New York. The book
concluded that it was "safer" to smoke cigarets having charcoal
filters, such as Liggett & Myers Tobacco Co.'s Lark brand. Several
industry sources, in fact, say the book amounts almost to a commercial for Lark.

Liggett & Myers denies, however, that it subsidized the book.
Hawthorn's chairman and president, W. Clement Stone, says,
"There are a lot of things that happened with that book that I
didn't approve of." He won't elaborate. Hawthorn agreed last
April to discontinue sales of the book after the deceptive practices
division of the Federal Trade Commission began investigating the
advertising.

A well-known Washington journalist reports that she was
approached last year by a tobacco industry representative and
asked if she would put her name on an article attacking the Surgeon General's report on smoking and health. The article already
had been written; the plan was to submit it to a national magazine
for which she writes frequently. The journalist, who asks not to be
identified, refused.

Several aspects of the True episode are in dispute. Charles N.
Barnard, True executive editor, denies that the magazine pro-

duced the reprints. However, they bore a note signed "The Editors" with no other attribution, and a True production official says they were printed on the True presses.

The production official says Tiderock, the public relations agency, ordered 607,000 copies. In addition, five tobacco companies say they bought a total of 449,000 copies from True. Mr. Barnard denies, however, that True got payments from any industry sources.

The promotional ads for the True article were paid for by individual tobacco companies through Tiderock, according to Reginald B. Wells, executive vice president of the agency. Mr. Wells says Tiderock is exploring various ways "to get the tobacco industry's side before the public."

The tobacco industry reported record sales and profits last year, but per capita consumption of cigarets declined for the first year since the Surgeon General's report was issued in 1964.

TRUE MAGAZINE AND THE CIGARETTE INDUSTRY

A comment from The American Cancer Society

Physicians, lawyers, school teachers, and many others have received copies of a magazine article claiming that "there is absolutely no proof that smoking causes human cancer."

The article appeared originally in *True* magazine and is entitled "To Smoke or Not to Smoke—That Is Still the Question." The author is Stanley Frank, now (but not when he wrote the article) employed by Hill and Knowlton, one of the public relations firms for the Tobacco Institute.

There seem to be several mailings: open ones to their stockholders by tobacco companies and an immense distribution to opinion leaders which purports to come from the Editors of *True*. There is no reference in the second mailing to a cigarette industry source or to any of the several known publicity agents of the cigarette industry.

We had wondered who was paying the many thousands of dollars for this expensive reprint, for the lists of addresses of opinion leaders, for the first-class postage.

Now the American Cancer Society congratulates the *Wall Street Journal* for exposing the real source of this devious mailing. It comes, according to the *Journal*, from Tiderock Corp., a second of the public relations firms employed by the Tobacco Institute. What is presented as a mailing to community leaders by the Editors of *True* is now exposed as a massive propaganda effort by the tobacco industry.

The article opens and closes with the Strickman Filter and speaks of Columbia University's "impressive" sponsorship. Aside from the reference to the Strickman Filter which Columbia has of course now dropped entirely, the article might have been written in 1965 (and may well have been since there is no other current data). The article ignores the Public Health Service report of 1967, "The Health Consequences of Smoking," which is based on 2,000 additional studies since 1964.

Why is this being given this handsome layout, rich paper, and massive distribution to opinion leaders?

Perhaps because it wraps up in lively journalese the tobacco industry's long time effort to merchandise doubt, to give cigarette smokers the impression that a major scientific controversy rages over whether cigarettes are harmful, that "only statistics" indict cigarette smoking as an extraordinarily dangerous habit.

Controversy there is—on the one hand is the tobacco industry and now its apologists in *True* magazine, on the other hand a vast body of scientists and physicians. So strong is the evidence against cigarettes that half of the physicians who once smoked cigarettes have kicked the habit (100,000 says the Public Health Service). And Congress has recognized the problem by requiring a warning on all cigarette packages.

The article's propaganda lines are familiar to those who have followed the releases and speeches from the tobacco industry.[1] In such form, where the source is known, the self interest of those distributing the material can be taken into account. However, presented in a general circulation magazine that has been respected in the past, and distributed allegedly by the Editors of the magazine as a factual piece dealing with controversy, this article may well mislead the unwary or inexperienced reader.

Thus, Mr. Frank wants the reader to feel that the famous Report of the Advisory Committee to the Surgeon General was in fact Dr. Luther Terry's creation. "Dr. Terry was in a tough spot," he writes, likening him to a district attorney who had to solve a murder. Actually the report was the result of more than a year's study by a most impartial group of scientists, half smokers, half not, selected only after both voluntary health agencies and the tobacco industry had been given a veto over their choice. (Because of the importance of this committee, we are listing its members' names at the end of this statement.) The report is, then, not just from Dr. Terry, nor the Public Health Service, but a reflection of the opinion and concern of the scientific community.

Mr. Frank makes the amazing statement that the Surgeon General's advisory committee "had reservations about the conclusions

---

[1] An article strikingly similar to this in propaganda line and content has just appeared in the National Enquirer, a sensational tabloid. Did the Enquirer lift from True or did both articles rely on generous tobacco industry sources? Both are equally misleading (see p. 218).

reached by Dr. Terry in the report." To the best of our knowledge this is utterly false. The only example of a reservation cited in the article is attributed to Dr. John B. Hickam, but in a formal letter to the House Committee on Commerce (which Mr. Frank conveniently ignores), Dr. Hickam wrote that he was in complete agreement with the Report.

There has been an interesting, personal development in the life of a committee member that is worth reporting: Louis F. Fieser, Ph.D., Sheldon Emery Professor of Chemistry, Harvard University, developed lung cancer and other diseases a year after the study and told of his experience in the *Reader's Digest*, "Early diagnosis, preoperative medical treatment, strict abstention from smoking and skillful surgery had pulled me through. . . . My case teaches two important lessons. The first one is the folly of saying 'It's probably too late to quit now.' I quit at a very late date but it was still in time. Suffering from emphysema, bronchitis, and worsened heart, I was very probably headed for death. But removal of the cause of these conditions—cigarette smoking in my case—stopped the degenerative processes and allowed nature, an extraordinarily powerful ally when given a chance, to start repairing the damage."

Mr. Frank presents a small carefully selected roster of individuals in science and medicine who claim that the case against the cigarette is unproved, or reject the harmfulness of cigarette smoking entirely. By so doing, he gives the impression that the scientific community is seriously divided in judgment. He fails to note that his "sources" constitute a minority—and an extremely small minority, at that—among those who have considered the question.

The United States Public Health Service, the American Cancer Society, the American Heart Association, the American Public Health Association, the Royal College of Physicians in England, and a host of other voluntary health organizations here and abroad have considered the evidence, in many cases have worked to produce the evidence through investigation, and are convinced that the cigarette is a distinct menace to health and life itself. The American Medical Association has indicted cigarette smoking as "a serious health hazard."

Further, when Mr. Frank states that the evidence against the cigarette is "only statistical" in nature, he is guilty of a double error: (1) He errs in matter of fact; and (2) he shows little if any understanding of the validity of statistics.

In 1960, the American Cancer Society issued a statement in which it said: ". . . clinical, epidemiological (population group), experimental, chemical, and pathological evidence presented by many studies . . . indicates beyond reasonable doubt that cigarette smoking is the major cause of the unprecedented increase in lung cancer."

Over the intervening years, the evidence—of all types—has grown both in magnitude and in conviction.

In several instances, Mr. Frank's assertions concerning scientific evidence can be shown to be flatly incorrect. When he states that, and repeats at the end of the article, "Long exposure to concentrated cigarette smoke *never* [Mr. Frank's emphasis] has produced lung cancer in an experimental animal . . ." he is trapped by the march of research.

Unfortunately for Mr. Frank, he has missed the eloquently titled article by R. J. C. Harris and G. Negroni in the *British Medical Journal* of December, 1967, "Production of Lung Carcinomas in C57BL Mice Exposed to a Cigarette Smoke and Air Mixture." Lung cancer *has* been produced in a series of experimental animals —and the C57BL mouse strain is one which (in the words of the authors) has apparently "a predominant gene for resistance to the induction of lung tumours." (Preliminary reports of this finding appeared in London six months earlier: a careful study of the literature might have led *True* to qualify rather drastically its author's repeated statement.)

Dr. Oscar Auerbach of the United States Veterans Administration, and colleagues have also gone a long way in demonstration of the harm wrought by the cigarette. In a series of biological—not "statistical"—experiments, Dr. Auerbach has shown that dogs in his laboratory which have been taught to smoke in roughly human fashion have demonstrated an appalling knack for the lung disease which in human beings would be termed "emphysema": a disease which in the decade from 1953 to 1963 increased in America some fivefold times. Furthermore, Dr. Auerbach reported "that histologic changes in bronchial epithelium, including dysplastic lesions, can be produced experimentally in animals exposed to cigarette smoke." (*JAMA*, Vol. 199, No. 4, January 23, 1967, pages 241–246; *Cancer*, Vol. 20, No. 12, December, 1967, pages 2055–2066.)

The evidence is far from being, as Mr. Frank would have his readers believe, "merely" statistical. Indeed, even if scientific findings *were* restricted to the results of population (epidemiological) studies—and they are not—they would not lack for validity. In denigrating "statistics," Mr. Frank appears to demonstrate something himself: a surprising ignorance of the fact that, properly used and interpreted, statistics are one of the most powerful tools in the scientific armamentarium.

Physicians know that essentially all important conclusions in the field of science, medicine, health, economics and business are based on statistics. It is through statistics that we know vaccinations prevent polio, smallpox, tetanus, diphtheria; that antibiotics cure many bacterial infections; that the pasteurization of milk and purification of water prevent many diseases.

Two recent examples of conclusions based entirely upon human statistical observations are the relation of the drug Thalidomide, taken by women in pregnancy, to the birth of deformed babies, and the risk of developing paralysis—estimated at less than one in 1,000,000—from the use of Type III oral poliomyelitis vaccine.

To refute each and every one of the errors in "To Smoke or Not to Smoke—That Is Still the Question" would require many pages. As can already be seen, Mr. Frank handles matter of fact and suggestion with a cheerful abandon which suggest the techniques of propaganda rather than true (or should it be *True*) expositional prose.

Here are a few of the exaggerations, absurdities, and errors:

1. "The cause of cancer is unknown," he writes—many causes of cancer are known and measures have been introduced successfully to prevent the disease: arsenic, lubricating oils formerly used in the textile industry, chimney soot, sun's rays, x-rays, to name a few of many known causes of cancer, *and now cigarettes*. The way to prevent most lung cancer is to stop smoking cigarettes.

2. "It is an established principle that a factor thought to be responsible for a disease must be found in all cases of it—and cancer strikes a dozen sites in the body not remotely associated with smoking." Apparently Mr. Frank is saying that since cigarettes do not cause all kinds of cancer, they cannot cause lung cancer. Mr. Frank's "established principle" is preposterous. Physicians recognize that cancer (called a host of diseases) in different sites will often have different causes.

3. Mr. Frank cites a source suggesting that lung cancer has not really skyrocketed in recent decades, but rather that techniques of diagnosis have improved. This would be a comforting thought, save for one thing: why, if cancer diagnostic means have improved so, have not other forms of cancer—particularly uterine cancer, for which we have the Pap test—shown a similar increase?

Mr. Frank says, "Since 1914, cigarette consumption in the United States has increased two-hundredfold, but the incidence of lung cancer has not increased nearly that much." The real figures are as follows: Since 1914, per capita cigarette smoking has increased seventeen times, whereas lung cancer mortality has increased thirty-two times (from 0.7 per 100,000 to 22.7 per 100,000—not, as Mr. Frank says later, 26.6). In lung cancer, mortality and incidence rates are unfortunately about the same.

4. Mr. Frank claims as one of his chief witnesses Dr. Joseph Berkson, and says, "The Cancer Bulletin, an official publication of the American Cancer Society, has referred to him as 'the acknowledged Dean of American Medical Statisticians.' " If Mr. Frank checks his facts he will find that *The Cancer Bulletin* is a publication of the M.D. Anderson Hospital and Tumor Institute in Texas, entirely independent of the American Cancer Society.

5. One of the oddest items in the article is the discussion of air pollution as a possible cause of lung cancer. Saying that this is not a new theory, the writer remarks, "In 1775 a London surgeon, Percival Potts, reported a high incidence of cancer among chimney sweeps." He did indeed, but the cancer was in the scrotum not the lung, and it was not caused by air pollution but by contact with coal tars.

6. "Inhaling should induce lung cancer if cigarettes are hazardous. Not a scrap of evidence has been found to corroborate the theory." False. See the reports of the Society's Cancer Prevention Study which demonstrate very clearly that inhaling is indeed hazardous. (Hammond, E. C., "Smoking in Relation to the Death Rates of One Million Men and Women." National Cancer Institute, Monograph 19, January, 1966.)

7. "Further, there is no proof that the chances of getting cancer are reduced by giving up smoking." False. Death rates in those

who stop smoking cigarettes drop rather rapidly as compared with those who continue smoking. Ten years after giving up cigarettes, death rates of smokers tend to approach those of persons who have never smoked regularly. (Hammond, E. C., "Smoking in Relation to the Death Rates of One Million Men and Women." National Cancer Institute, Monograph 19, January, 1966.)

8. Mr. Frank doesn't seem to know that the mortality rate for lung cancer in women has risen 400 percent since 1930 (from 1.5 per 100,000 to 6.4 per 100,000). He makes the extraordinary statement, "There has been a tremendous increase in women smokers during the last generation but their death rate from lung cancer had remained almost steady."

Despite the propaganda of the cigarette industry, cigarette smoking has been established as most hazardous.

We would remind cigarette smokers that:

Men aged 25 who have never smoked regularly can expect over six and a half years more of life than men who smoke one pack or more a day. Of men aged 25, twice as many of the heavy cigarette smokers as of the nonsmokers die before 65 years of age.

Every regular cigarette smoker is injured, though not in the same degree. Cigarette smoking kills some, makes others lung cripples, gives still others far more than their share of illness and loss of work days. Cigarette smoking is not a gamble: all regular cigarette smokers studied at autopsy show the effects.

At first, the American Cancer Society felt it best to ignore *True's* article. Given the irresponsibility of the research, its ambiguous status as a "fact article," and its fantastically wide reprint distribution to such opinion leaders as physicians, lawyers, and teachers, the Society felt the need to reply and to raise the question as to the wisdom and morality of the distribution of this misleading article from a carefully concealed tobacco industry source.

Does this indicate that the Tobacco Institute, which has usually been quite candid now feels guilty or is running scared?

What do Governor Meyner and the industry code authority think of this deceptive promotion?

How do the Editors of *True* justify their covering note?

Advisory committee on smoking and health
to the surgeon general

We think it worthwhile to remind readers just who was on the Advisory Committee, their positions at the time of the study, and their fields of specialty:

Stanhope Bayne-Jones, M.D., LL.D. (Retired), Former Dean, Yale School of Medicine (1935–40), former President, Joint Administrative Board, Cornell University, New York Hospital Medical Center (1947–52); former President, Society of American Bacteriologists (1929), and American Society of Pathology and Bacteriology (1940). Field: Nature and Causation of Disease in Human Populations. Dr. Bayne-Jones served also as a special consultant to the Committee staff.

Walter J. Burdette, M.D., Ph.D., Head of Department of Surgery, University of Utah School of Medicine, Salt Lake City. Fields: Clinical & Experimental Surgery; Genetics.

William G. Cochran, M.A., Professor of Statistics, Harvard University. Field: Mathematical Statistics, with Special Application to Biological Problems.

Emmanuel Farber, M.D., Ph.D., Chairman, Department of Pathology, University of Pittsburgh. Field: Experimental and Clinical Pathology.

Louis F. Fieser, Ph.D., Sheldon Emory Professor of Organic Chemistry, Harvard University. Field: Chemistry of Carcinogenic Hydrocarbons.

Jacob Furth, M.D., Professor of Pathology, Columbia University, and Director of Pathology Laboratories, Francis Delafield Hospital, New York, N.Y. Field: Cancer Biology.

John B. Hickam, M.D., Chairman, Department of Internal Medicine, University of Indiana, Indianapolis. Fields: Internal Medicine, Physiology of Cardiopulmonary Disease.

Charles LeMaistre, M.D., Professor of Internal Medicine, The University of Texas Southwestern Medical School, and Medical Director, Woodlawn Hospital, Dallas, Texas. Fields: Internal Medicine, Pulmonary Diseases, Preventive Medicine.

Leonard M. Schuman, M.D., Professor of Epidemiology, University of Minnesota School of Public Health, Minneapolis. Field: Health and Its Relationship to the Total Environment.

Maurice H. Seevers, M.D., Ph.D., Chairman, Department of Pharmacology, University of Michigan, Ann Arbor. Field: Pharmacology of Anesthesia and Habit-Forming Drugs.

IF YOU WANT TO GIVE UP CIGARETTES

APPENDIX D

If you want to give up cigarettes: Congratulations!

This pamphlet seeks to round up helpful suggestions from experimental projects that have been carefully evaluated. No sure techniques are offered, no absolute laws of human behavior provided. There are different kinds of smokers and what helps one may not work with another. Individuals must choose for themselves from what is presented here.

Each man (and woman) makes a personal decision on the important matter of smoking cigarettes. The fact that you are reading this pamphlet indicates that you are properly concerned.*

Many millions have given up cigarette smoking. Although for some people it is surprisingly easy to quit, most find it rather difficult. Psychologists estimate that half of all cigarette smokers can stop without too much difficulty once they make up their minds to try. They feel only minor or temporary discomfort. Others suffer intensely, almost unbearably for days and weeks. Remember that those who have tried to stop a number of times may succeed this time.

Will you really make the effort? We hope so.

THE AMERICAN CANCER SOCIETY

* Copies of Clifton R. Read's attractive illustrated booklet, from which this Appendix is taken, are available from local units of the American Cancer Society.

This pamphlet developed out of discussions at a two-day conference called by the American Cancer Society on withdrawal programs and cigarette smoking. Participating, and contributing ideas and materials, but not responsible for the content selected here, were Borje E. V. Ejrup, M.D., Clinical Associate Professor of Medicine, Director, Anti-Smoking Clinic, The New York Hospital Cornell Medical Center, New York, N.Y.; Donald T. Fredrickson, M.D., Director, Smoking Control Program, New York City Department of Health; Judith S. Mausner, M.D., Assistant Professor of Epidemiology, Department of Preventive Medicine, Woman's Medical College, Philadelphia, Pa.; Bernard Mausner, Ph.D., Professor of Psychology, Chairman, Department of Psychology, Beaver College, Glenside, Pa.; Charles A. Ross, M.D., Chief, Department of Thoracic Surgery, Roswell Park Memorial Institute, Buffalo, New York; David Sharp, M.D., Medical Consultant, National Clearinghouse for Smoking and Health, United States Public Health Service, Arlington, Va.; and Jerome L. Schwartz, Dr. P. H., Project Director, Smoking Control Research Project, Berkeley, California. We have also drawn on ideas from others including Donald Pumroy, Ph.D., Counselling Center, University of Maryland, and Silvan Tomkins, Ph.D., Center for Research in Cognition and Affect, City University of New York, and a member of the American Cancer Society's Committee on Tobacco and Cancer. Representing the American Cancer Society were Harold S. Diehl, M.D., at that time Deputy Executive Vice President for Research and Medical Affairs; Walter James, Vice President for Public Education, and Clifton R. Read, Senior Editor-Consultant.

Once you have stopped

If you are like most cigarette smokers, you will in two weeks or less say farewell to that hacking, shattering morning cough, good-by to ugly thick phlegm, adios to smoker's headaches and unpleasant cigarette-induced mouth and stomach complaints.

You will be saving—how much? Well, how much do you smoke up in dollars every week? Could be considerable.

You will no longer burn cigarette holes in clothing, furniture, rugs, or tablecloths. (The National Fire Protection Association says that "smoking and matches" caused a property loss of $80,400,000 in 1965.)

Food will tend to taste better and your sense of smell will return to normal.

Cigarette breath (it can be very offensive) will disappear.

Q Day, cigarette quitting day, might well be renamed K Day— kindness day for both you and your friends.

By quitting cigarettes you are instituting an immediate program of kindness to your lungs, your heart, your stomach, your nose, your throat.

A garland of facts

Since you have decided to give up cigarette smoking, you probably know the risks of the habit. However, a brief selection from the mountains of facts that have developed through research, published since 1954, may be useful.

Not a gamble

Cigarette smoking used to be compared to Russian roulette. Now we know better. Every regular cigarette smoker is injured, though not in the same degree. Cigarette smoking kills some, makes others lung cripples, gives still others far more than their share of illness and loss of work days. Cigarette smoking is not a gamble: regular cigarette smokers studied at autopsy all show the effects.

The more cigarettes, the more cancer of the lung

The regular cigarette smoker runs a risk of death from lung cancer ten times greater than the nonsmoker, men who smoke more than a pack a day have about 20 times as much lung cancer as non-smokers have. Unfortunately, early diagnosis of lung cancer is very difficult: only about one in 20 cases is cured.

Six and one-half years, 78 months, 23,725 days

Men aged 25 who have never smoked regularly can expect six-and-a-half years more of life than men who smoke *one* pack or more a day. Twice as many heavy smokers (two packs a day) will die between 25 and 65 years of age, as nonsmokers.

Those minutes of life

The average heavy smoker (two or more packs a day) smokes about three-quarters of a million cigarettes during his lifetime. As a result, he loses about 4.4 million minutes—8.3 years—of life compared with nonsmokers. This amounts to a loss of almost six minutes per cigarette smoked: a minute of life for a minute of smoking.

Give your heart a break

Male smokers (10 or more cigarettes a day) between 45 and 54 have more than three times the death rate from heart attacks that nonsmokers do. In the ages between 40 and 64, heart attacks prematurely kill some 45,000 cigarette smoking men.

How to escape work

Cigarette smokers between 45 and 64 miss 50 percent more days at work than do nonsmokers. Or, to say it another way: According to the Public Health Service, if cigarette smokers had the same rates of illness as nonsmokers, some 77 million working days would not be lost annually.

A *deep breath*

Emphysema, a relatively rare disease a few years ago, is now a major cause of medical disability in this country. Most emphysema is caused by cigarette smoking. The disease is both a crippler and a killer causing the lungs to lose their elasticity. Eventually the effort to breathe becomes a constant, agonizing struggle.

Live a little more

A longer and healthier life is high on our priorities: giving up cigarette smoking is the most important action that the average individual can take that will improve the physical quality of his daily life, extend his life expectancy, and increase his chances of avoiding lung cancer, heart disease, emphysema and a number of other nasty complaints.

Some of the millions who make it

(The following brief sketches are based on fact from letters, conversations, reports but with names and details altered. They have been selected with the intention of helping others to go and do likewise.)

William is a psychiatrist who decided soon after the Report of the Advisory Committee to the Surgeon General that he ought to stop cigarettes. What triggered his actual decision? He suspects it was a morning cough, but he is not sure! In any case, he stopped and reports that he watched television for several evenings (which he rarely did), ate rather more often than was his custom, did some strenuous skiing, and was happy that his wife cleared the house at once of all cigarettes and ashtrays. He was uncomfortable for a few

days, but not climbing any walls. He hasn't smoked for three
years.

Joan is a writer who reads seriously. After the Surgeon General's
Report she stopped smoking cigarettes. Cold turkey. No gum, no
candy, no gaining of weight. Some bad temper for a few days but
it was not a big or difficult deal.

Pete is a carpenter who smoked two packs a day for 25 years. He
was proud, however, that his three sons did not smoke. He wanted
to quit but was hooked, he knew it, and he told his boys never to
take up the habit. When they believed and obeyed him, he was
delighted. He stopped only after an operation in which two-thirds
of his stomach was taken out because of an ulcer. He still doesn't
discuss the fact that he has given up smoking but he hasn't
smoked for a year and he was in the hospital long enough so that
when he went back on the job and people began offering him a
smoke, he was able to say "no" very calmly.

John was a brilliantly successful advertising man who smoked two
packs of cigarettes a day: when he began to cough, and this happened half a dozen times in a work day, it took him embarrassed
moments to get over it. He had thought of stopping cigarettes,
even made half-hearted trials—but at last he decided to go for
broke. His first step was to keep a careful record of when he
smoked each cigarette, and how much he wanted it. Then he
selected a future Q Day and told his family and friends what he
was doing. He began to cut down, 50 percent each week for four
weeks, and he laid in mints and gum.

When Q Day arrived he stopped. It was a rough experience and
at one time he was in such a serious depression that he frightened
his wife. After a visit to his physician, however, he stood by his
decision. During the first three months he gained 15 pounds, but
he lost all of this later, his cough is gone, and he feels a hundred
percent better. He hasn't smoked a cigarette for two years.

George is a television announcer who never smoked on camera. But, during his tense, challenging work, he consumed more than two packs of cigarettes a day. Finally, he and a lawyer friend bet each other $1,000 that each could stay off cigarettes longer than the other. They deposited the money in a special bank account and agreed that after 18 months they would take the money and go to Europe. Neither has smoked for six months. George found that he couldn't sleep, that his food didn't taste any better and that he passionately hated all cigarette advertising. But George was Scotch and he wasn't out to lose one thousand dollars. His bad time lasted for almost four weeks—now he is convinced that he will never smoke again.

Linda reports she really puffed away at cigarettes when she was worried or tense. She was disturbed by stories of the risks of smoking and wished she could stop but continued until (she says) one of the American Cancer Society's announcements gave her just the push she needed. That was three months ago, about the same time her husband lost his job, her four year old child broke her arm, her baby had his first nasty cold. Linda wrote the Society that despite all the tensions she "came through with a smile and a prayer, but no cigarette."

Harold—a reporter of considerable distinction—smoked three packs a day: at the typewriter, before and after breakfast, during lunch, in the afternoon and evening. Any tests would have shown him as a thoroughly convinced smoker, a bad risk for a withdrawal program. However, he stopped, cold turkey, and has not smoked for 10 years. Why? His specialty was science writing and he decided that if the scientists he trusted were right he was a fool to go on smoking. For two weeks he was in considerable discomfort, but with gum and candy he kept going. He says he feels great since he stopped smoking.

There are nineteen million ex-cigarette smokers in the United States: about one in five adult men in this country has dropped the habit. Those who give up cigarettes report a great sense of satisfaction, of tremendous pride in being able to do it. To learn a new way of living, a way without cigarette smoking, is very rewarding to the ego—and to the ego's mate. *You can kick the habit!*

As you approach Q Day

Many stress willpower as the decisive factor in giving up cigarettes. For them the sense that they can manage their own lives is of great importance. They enjoy challenging themselves and, with an effort of will, they break the cigarette habit.

Thus, some psychologists describe stopping cigarettes as an exercise in self-mastery, one that introduces a new dimension of self-control.

Others, often successful in many aspects of living, find that willpower does not help them in giving up cigarettes. They try to stop, they do not, and they feel guilty over their weakness. This is a mistake, since many smokers fail in their first and second, even their fifth attempts and then finally succeed. Those whose "will" fails in breaking the habit are not weak but different. Their approach must be less through determination and more through relearning new behavior with patience and perseverance.

Self-suggestion, when one is relaxed, aimed at changing one's feelings and thoughts about cigarettes can be useful.

One health educator remarked recently, "nothing succeeds like will power and a little blood in the sputum."

To think of stopping smoking as self-denial is an error: the ex-smoker should not believe that he is giving up an object of value, however dependent he may be on it. If he begins to feel sorry for himself and broods on his sufferings, they may well become more severe and indeed unendurable. He must recognize that he is teaching himself a more positive, more constructive, more reward-ing behavior.

Try cutting down

An important first step in the process of giving up cigarettes for many smokers is to set the date for Q Day, when you are going to stop completely and, as it approaches, to gradually reduce the number of cigarettes you smoke, day by day, or week by week.

A good system is to decide only to smoke once an hour—or to stop smoking between the hours of 9 and 10 o'clock, 11 and 12, 1 and 2, 3 and 4, etc. And then to extend the nonsmoking time by half an hour, an hour, two hours.

You may decide to halve the cigarettes you smoke week by week, giving yourself four weeks to Q Day.

How about smoking only half of each cigarette?

In the process of reducing the number of daily cigarettes, try various possibilities; if you have one pocket in which you always carry your pack, put it in another so that you will have to fumble for it. If you always use your right hand to bring your cigarette to your mouth, use the left hand. Is it your custom to rest the ciga-rette in the right corner of the mouth? Try the left side.

Make it a real effort to get a cigarette:

Wrap your package in several sheets of paper or place it in a tightly covered box. If you leave your change at home you won't be able to use a cigarette machine.

Shift from cigarettes you like to an unpalatable brand.

Before you light up, ask yourself "Do I really want this cigarette or am I just acting out of empty habit?"

A smoker may find an unlighted cigarette in the mouth is helpful. Others enjoy handling and playing with a cigarette.

Cigarette smoking is a habit that is usually very well learned—learning the habit of not smoking can be difficult. It can help in breaking into your habit chain to make yourself aware of the nature and frequency of your smoking behavior.

Keep a track record

Many smokers have found that a useful step in understanding their smoking is the keeping of a daily record on a card like that opposite.

In your gradual withdrawal you may decide to eliminate those daily cigarettes that you find are rated over 6 on the scale, i.e., ones you want very little.

Or you may wish to give up first the cigarettes you like most. In any case keeping a smoking log will give you information about yourself, make you more aware of what your smoking habits are.

You may find that you are largely a social smoker, that smoking makes you feel closer to others, more welcome at a party, that you seem to have more friends. A cigarette may play a surprisingly large part in your picture of yourself as a mature and successful man.

How do you convince yourself that people like and respect you for more important reasons than your cigarette? Try going without a cigarette and see.

Plus and minus

Write down carefully, after some thought, in one column the reasons why you smoke and in another all the reasons why you should give up cigarettes.

DAILY RECORD

Monday, A.M.   Check on scale
(Enter time   Wanted cigarette
cigarette smoked)   Wanted cigarette   very little
                     very much

_____   1   2   3   4   5   6   7

_____   1   2   3   4   5   6   7

Monday, P.M.

_____   1   2   3   4   5   6   7

As you turn this exercise over in your mind, new material will occur to you for one or the other columns. Thoughtful concentration on your reasons for giving up cigarettes is important in changing your behavior.

Four smoking styles

Dr. Silvan Tomkins distinguishes four general types of smoking behavior. An abbreviated summary of the types follows:

Habitual smoking   Here the smoker may hardly be aware that he has a cigarette in his mouth. He smokes as if it made him feel good, or feel better, but in fact it does neither. He may once have regarded smoking as an important sign of status. But now smoking is automatic. The habitual smoker who wants to give up must first become aware of when he is smoking. Knowledge of the pattern of his smoking is a first step towards change.

Positive affect smoking   Here smoking seems to serve as a stimulant that produces exciting pleasure, or is used as a relaxant, to heighten enjoyment, as at the end of a meal. Here a youngster demonstrates his manhood or his defiance of his parents. This smoker may enjoy most the handling of a cigarette or the sense and sight of smoke curling out of his mouth. If these smokers can be persuaded to make an effort, they may find giving up cigarettes relatively painless.

Negative affect smoking This is sedative smoking, using the habit to reduce feelings of distress, fear, shame, or disgust or any combination of them. This person may not smoke at all when things go well, on vacation, or at a party, but under tension, when things go badly, at the office or at home, he reaches for a cigarette. These smokers give up often, but when the heat and pressure of the day hit them, when there's a challenge, they find it very hard to resist a cigarette. A strong substitute, like nibbling ginger root, may be useful.

Addictive smoking The smoker is always aware when he is not smoking. The absence of a cigarette is uncomfortably obvious. The lack of a cigarette builds need, desire, and discomfort at not smoking. With this increasing need is the expectation that a cigarette will reduce discomfort—and the cigarette does give relief—for a moment. Pleasure at smoking is real, just as the buildup of discomfort at not smoking is real, sometimes rapid and intolerable. The enjoyment of the cigarette, however, is very brief, and may be disappointing—but the suffering for lack of even slight relief is considerable. For this smoker, tapering off doesn't seem to work: the only solution is to quit cold: once you have been through the intense pain of breaking your psychological addiction, you are unlikely to start smoking again. The experience of giving up has been too uncomfortable—and too memorable for you to risk having to go through it again.

Some such smokers have found it useful to increase during the week before Q Day the number of cigarettes smoked, to go from two packs to four packs, to force yourself to smoke so that your body will be in actual revolt against the double dose of tar and nicotine.

For information on a Smoker's Self-Testing Kit (four questionnaires, etc., to help one to understand personal reasons for, and style of, smoking) write to the National Clearinghouse for Smoking and Health, United States Public Health Service, 4040 North Fairfax Drive, Arlington, Va., 22203.

The week before Q Day

Think over your list of reasons why you should not smoke: the risk of disease, the blurring of the taste of food, the cost, the cough, the bad breath, the mess and smell of morning-after ashtrays.

Concentrate each evening when you are relaxed, just before you fall asleep, on one dreadful result of cigarette smoking. Repeat and repeat and repeat that single fact. Drive home another fact the next night and another the next.

Review the facts that you know about the risks of cigarette smoking. Remind yourself that there, but for the grace of God, go you; that you may indeed, if you continue smoking, lose six and a half years of life; that—if you are a heavy smoker—your chances of dying between 25 and 65 years of age are twice as great as those of the nonsmoker. Are the six minutes of pleasure in a cigarette worth six fewer minutes of life to a heavy smoker? Would you fly in an airplane if the chances of crash and death were even close to the risks of cigarette smoking? Think over why it is that 100,000 physicians have quit cigarette smoking.

Action: Q Day

Let us suppose that you know, now, when and where and how you smoke. You have suggested again and again to your tired mind that smoking is a dangerous business.

"But what will I do the morning of Q Day when, mind or no mind, I desperately want a cigarette?"

We hope you will prove that you are stronger than your dependence. Here are some tips * that may prove useful when you have an impulse to smoke!

For the mouth   Drink frequent glasses of water.

Nibble fruit, cookies, eat somewhat self-pleasing food.

Suck candy mints and/or chew gum (sugarless gum will be easier on your teeth).

Chew bits of fresh ginger when you start to reach for a cigarette. (Take this gently, ginger root is aromatic and pervasive—some experience it as burning, others as clean and satisfying.)

Bite a clove.

Nicotine replacement   Lobeline sulphate tablets, available without prescription, make it easier for many people to stop cigarettes. Authorities disagree as to whether they provide a substitute that will help satisfy your body's craving for nicotine! Try them out.

(Since some individuals—those with stomach ulcers, for instance —should not use these tablets, it will be wiser to check with your physician.)

Be vigorous: exercise   Strenuous physical activity that demands effort and keeps you busy can be very helpful.

Vacation is a good time for some people to stop: camping, mountain climbing, tennis.

* Our preferred definition for "tip": "A useful hint or idea." These are not scientifically proved. Many people have found one or another of them helpful.

Stretching exercises or long walks can be relaxing.

Go *"no smoking"* For a few days, spend as much time as possible in libraries or other places where smoking is forbidden. Ride in "No Smoking" cars.

A spurt of motion picture or theater-going will pass many hours.

Keep away from friends who are heavy smokers for two weeks.

Use your lungs Deep breaths of air can be wonderfully calming.

Inhalers—that reduce nasal stuffiness—may help tide you over the first few days.

After meals For some the cigarette after breakfast coffee, at the end of lunch or dinner, is most important. Instead of a cigarette try a mouth wash after each meal.

If you have had a specific pattern that you have followed after dinner you may want to change it: read a book instead of a newspaper, skip familiar television programs, sit in another comfortable chair, try crossword puzzles or take care of some household task you have been putting off, take your dog out for a walk.

Reward yourself Be sure you have your favorite food on Q Day.

Give yourself all the things that you like best—except cigarettes.

When you have saved a bit of money by not smoking, buy yourself a present: perhaps a new record, or a blouse, or necktie, or book or a trinket.

On the other hand you may prefer to do all the things that are familiar and comfortable for you and to which you are used— except to smoke cigarettes. Take your choice.

So—now you are on your own

When the impulse to smoke is strong, try a substitute: a drink of water, a piece of gum, a walk around the block, stretching and breathing.

These substitutes may only satisfy you temporarily—but they will keep you alert and aware and will soften the strength of your desire to smoke. Equally important are constant reminders to yourself of why you are stopping cigarettes. Remember the reasons that you put down for not smoking? Recall the basic data about disease, disability, and death that are caused by cigarettes.

You may be very uncomfortable but "this too shall pass" relates also to cigarette-less shakes, irritation and temper, the urge to climb walls, depression, anxiety. Time is a great healer.

A minority of cigarette smokers go through the terrors of the damned after they quit. Even these—when they come on the fresh air side—report great pride at having been able to give up.

Unfortunately, fear of failure to make it seems to deter very many men and women from even trying—but for many, giving up cigarettes, while uncomfortable and a strain, is by no means agony. After all their terrible expectations, stopping can seem relatively easy.

Questions and answers

Do you believe in cold turkey quitting? Yes, for some, no, for others. If you are a really "addicted" smoker, psychologists favor the sudden, decisive break.

For some, gradual withdrawal is less painful and entirely satisfactory.

Some cigarette smokers shift to pipes and cigars—there is of course some risk of mouth cancer from these but over-all mortality of cigar and pipe smokers is only a little higher than among non-smokers, provided the smoke is not inhaled.

What about going to a cigarette withdrawal clinic for help? If there is a clinic or program in your community, you may find it useful. The American Cancer Society favors such efforts.

Sharing your withdrawal experiences with others and working with them on a common problem can be very helpful. The clinic may make it considerably easier in various ways to stop cigarette smoking.

However, remember, no clinic can provide a sure result. In this matter you must be both patient and physician.

Shall I make a big thing of Q Day? Some find it most satisfactory to work on a schedule in which Q Day, quitting day, is singled out as the important, decisive day in their personal lives—that indeed it is.

Others who have known for a long time that cigarettes are bad for them and that sooner or later they will stop, wake up one morning and say to themselves "This is it. No more cigarettes."

What motivates them? An obituary, an antismoking commercial on television, a magazine article, a leaflet brought home from school by a child, a worried look from their son, being fed up with a repeated cough. There are many possible stimuli to stop, but almost always beneath the casual-seeming but bold decision are months, often years of thought and worry.

What if I fail to make it? Don't be discouraged: many thousands who stopped did so only after several attempts.

Some people prefer to stop for just one day at a time. They promise themselves 24 hours of freedom from cigarettes and when the day is over they make a commitment to themselves for one more day. And another. And another. At the end of any 24-hour period they can go back to cigarettes without betraying themselves—but they usually do not.

Is smoking a real addiction? This depends on your definition of words. In any case, smokers obviously can become very strongly, very tragically dependent on cigarettes.

However, the discomfort that most feel at giving up cigarettes is not like the painful withdrawal symptoms that drug addicts report.

Giving up cigarettes is much closer to the discomfort and the irritation produced by dieting than to the agony of stopping a drug. As so many know, dieting in an effort to lose fifteen or twenty pounds can be a most uncomfortable experience—but when you have done it, you have a fine feeling.

Shall I throw out our ashtrays? One school of thought asks, do you leave a bottle of whiskey near an alcholic? Their recommendation is to get rid of cigarettes, ashtrays, anything that might remind a smoker of his former habit.

Others take a different view and even suggest carrying cigarettes to demonstrate to yourself that you can resist temptation. Choose for yourself.

Shall I tell others of my decision? Some do, some don't. Some find that the wider they spread the news of their decision the easier it is for them to make it stick. Others regard not smoking as their own personal business and keep it almost entirely to themselves. Will you strengthen your decision if your wife and friends know that you have committed yourself?

Will I gain weight?   Many do. Food is a substitute for cigarettes for many people. And your appetite may be fresher and stronger.

During the first few weeks of giving up cigarettes some psychologists recommend pampering yourself: eating well, drinking well, enjoying those things that are pleasant and fulfilling.

Some people, those to whom self-mastery is vital, get rewards out of controlling their wish for fattening food at the same time that they are licking the urge for cigarettes.

Again, it depends upon the person and his approach.

How about hypnosis?   This is unproven. Why not discuss the matter with a physician, if you are interested.

Shall I see my physician?   Yes. However, the problem is yours, not his, and he may not feel that he can be helpful. On the other hand he may be able to give you sympathetic support and may prescribe medication. He can be helpful, also, in suggesting a diet which will prevent you from gaining too much weight.

Physicians as a profession have been leaders in acting on the risks of cigarette smoking: the Public Health Service estimates that 100,000 physicians (half of the physicians who once were cigarette smokers) have kicked the habit. A California study shows that only 21.3 percent of all physicians in the state are cigarette smokers now.

Why do so many people smoke cigarettes?   Surely one reason is that the cigarette industry spends about $300,000,000 a year in promoting the habit and in challenging the facts that scientists have produced that point to the dangers of the habit.

Another reason is that something in cigarettes, probably nicotine, is habit forming: smokers become dependent rather rapidly on cigarettes.

Cigarette smoking is essentially a twentieth century habit, encouraged by wars, by brilliant advertising, and by the development of remarkably efficient automatic machinery that produces those millions of round, firmly packed cigarettes.

It is only within the last 15 years that we have learned, through research pioneered by the American Cancer Society, that this personal and socially accepted habit is extremely dangerous. Cigarette smoking is deeply embedded in our life: agriculture, industry, government, the communications media, all have a stake in it. It is still widely accepted, even though proven to be a most certain hazard to health.

Because promotion is important in maintaining the habit's popularity, the Society believes all cigarette advertising in all media should be terminated. We hope that this goal will be achieved voluntarily and that governmental action won't be necessary.

Approaches in giving up cigarette smoking

If you don't stop immediately and permanently:

1 List the reasons for and against smoking.
2 Select Q Day—change to low tar and nicotine cigarette.
3 Chart your smoking habits for at least two weeks: how many cigarettes, when, the most and least important.
4 Repeat each night, at least ten times, one of your reasons for not smoking cigarettes.
5 Eliminate one category of cigarettes: the most or the least desired.
6 Secure a supply of substitutes: mints, lobeline tablets, ginger root, etc.
7 Quit on Q Day—try the different substitutes as the wish to smoke recurs—enlist your wife or a friend in a busy series of events: eating well, going to the movies or theater, exercise and many long walks, moderate drinking.

8 If you are depressed, see your physician and discuss your symptoms.

9 Keep reminding yourself, again and again, of the shocking risks in cigarette smoking.

To smoke or not to smoke?

A story is told of two boys who knew a man who was supposed to be wise and were determined to challenge him. They caught a small bird and decided on a formula that they felt could not fail. They would go to the wise man with their hands cupped and say: "Tell us, wise man, is the bird, that one of us holds in his hands, alive or dead?" If he said "dead" they would release the bird. If he said "alive" a squeeze of the hands would prove him wrong. When they confronted him and asked the question, the wise man smiled, and considered, and finally said, "The answer is in your hands."

Books that may help you stop smoking

Herewith are names of several stimulating books that may be of interest and help to those wishing to stop cigarette smoking.

ALLEN, W. A., G. ANGERMAN, AND W. A. FACKLER: *Learning to Live without Cigarettes*, Philadelphia, Health Department, Room 540, 1967, 113 pp.

BREAN, HERBERT: *How to Stop Smoking*, Pocket Books Inc., New York (C439), 1963, 111 pp.

FOX-MARTIN, MILTON: *How to Give Up Smoking Without Gaining Weight*, Fox-Martin and Fox-Martin, 1966, 64 pp.

OCHSNER, ALTON: *Smoking and Your Life*, Julian Messner, Publishers, Inc., New York, 1964, 144 pp.

TAR AND NICOTINE CONTENT OF CERTAIN BRANDS OF CIGARETTES

APPENDIX E

CIGARETTES
CAUSE DISABILITY, DISEASE & DEATH!
★★★

IF YOU DO SMOKE CIGARETTES, YOU SHOULD KNOW THE RELATIVE AMOUNTS
OF NICOTINE AND TAR IN YOUR CIGARETTES, AS DETERMINED BY THE
FEDERAL TRADE COMMISSION.

THE LESS TAR & NICOTINE YOU INHALE THE BETTER!

CIGARETTE BRAND	TYPE	Nicotine content in mg.	Tar content in mg.	CIGARETTE BRAND	TYPE	Nicotine content in mg.	Tar content in mg.
MARVELS	Reg. Size, Filter	.12	3.9	KOOL	King Size, Filter Menthol	1.56	20.2
	King Size, Filter	.22	6.4		Reg. Size, Non Filter	1.84	26.3
	King Size, Non Filter	.82	21.8				
CARLTON	King Size, Filter	.50	7.2	MARLBORO	King Size, Filter (hard pk.)	1.34	20.4
CASCADE	King Size, Filter Menthol	.27	7.8		King Size, Filter	1.41	20.7
DUKE OF DURHAM	King Size, Filter	.38	10.4		100 mm, Filter	1.38	20.9
					King Size, Filter Menthol	1.72	24.4
TRUE	King Size, Filter Menthol	.68	12.7	WINSTON	King Size, Filter	1.29	20.4
	King Size, Filter	.65	12.8		King Size, Filter (hard pk.)	1.22	20.8
KING SANO & SANO	King Size, Filter	.38	12.9		100 mm, Filter Menthol	1.66	25.2
	King Size, Filter Menthol	.42	13.8		100 mm, Filter	1.74	26.7
	Reg. Size, Non Filter	.61	20.5				
DOMINO	King Size, Filter	.71	15.0	RALEIGH	King Size, Filter	1.53	20.8
PARLIAMENT	King Size, Filter (hard pk.)	1.01	15.8		King Size, Non Filter	1.98	27.8
	King Size, Filter	1.05	16.1	VICEROY	King Size, Filter	1.43	21.0
KENT	King Size, Filter	1.09	17.4		King Size, Filter (hard pk.)	1.43	21.4
	100 mm, Filter	1.46	23.4				
TAREYTON	King Size, Filter	1.07	17.5	CAMEL	King Size, Filter	1.26	21.0
	100 mm, Filter	1.23	20.2		Reg. Size, Non Filter	1.39	24.2
L & M	Reg. Size, Filter	.93	18.5	CHESTERFIELD	King Size, Filter Menthol	1.19	21.0
	King Size, Filter (hard pk.)	1.06	19.4		King Size, Filter	1.16	22.4
	King Size, Filter	1.15	21.3		Reg. Size, Non Filter	1.20	22.7
	100 mm, Filter Menthol	1.44	25.3		King Size, Non Filter	1.54	28.6
	100 mm, Filter	1.41	25.6				
PHILIP MORRIS	King Size, Filter	1.29	18.9	SALEM	King Size, Filter Menthol	1.36	21.1
	King Size, Filter Menthol	1.28	20.0		100 mm, Filter Menthol	1.74	27.0
	Reg. Size, Non Filter	1.45	22.7				
	King Size, Non Filter	1.79	28.1	PALL MALL	100 mm, Filter Menthol	1.47	22.3
LUCKY STRIKE	100 mm, Filter Menthol	1.03	19.4		100 mm, Filter	1.56	23.1
	100 mm, Filter	1.28	20.6		95 mm, Filter Menthol (hard pk.)	1.45	25.9
	King Size, Filter Menthol	1.22	20.7		King Size, Non Filter	1.60	27.1
	King Size, Filter	1.33	21.7		95 mm, Filter (hard pk.)	1.58	28.1
	Reg. Size, Non Filter	1.55	26.4				

Figures are as published by the FTC on November 20, 1967. The latest figures for all brands, as reported periodically by the Federal Trade Commission, are available free upon request from the National Clearinghouse for Smoking and Health, 4040 North Fairfax Drive, Arlington, Va. 22203, or from the Federal Trade Commission, Washington, D.C. (Courtesy American Cancer Society.)

GLOSSARY

addiction: a physiological dependence upon either a drug or a druglike substance

adeno: prefix meaning "relating to a gland"

adrenal glands: glands of internal secretions attached to upper portion of the kidneys

aneurism: a balloonlike enlargement of an artery, due to a weakening of the wall

angina pectoris: severe pain related to the heart; usually radiates down the left arm

apoplexy: a stroke

arteriole: a small artery

autopsy: dissection of a dead body to learn the cause, seat, or nature of disease, or the cause of death; a postmortem examination

benign: relatively harmless

benzpyrene: a cancer-producing chemical in tobacco smoke
biostatistics: statistical analysis of data relating to life
blood pressure: the pressure within an artery
blood pressure diastolic: the pressure between heartbeats
blood pressure systolic: the pressure during the heartbeat
bronchitis: inflammation of the lining of a bronchus
bronchogenic: originating in a bronchus
buccal cavity: the inside of the mouth
Buerger's disease: deficient circulation of arms, legs, hands, and feet
     due to the formation of a thrombus in an artery supplying the
     part with blood

cancer: a collection of body tissue cells which reproduce rapidly and
     without limit until they destroy life; a malignant tumor, which
     usually gives rise to secondary growths (metastases)
carbon dioxide: a gas containing one atom of carbon and two atoms
     of oxygen: produced in burning and breathing—not poisonous
carbon monoxide: a gas of one atom of carbon and one of oxygen:
     produced by burning with insufficient oxygen—very poisonous
carcinogen: a substance that will cause cancer
carcinoma: cancer arising from epithelial tissue
cholera: a highly fatal infection of the intestinal tract, usually trans-
     mitted by contaminated drinking water or food
cholesterol: a crystalline fatlike substance found in all animal fats and
     in bile, blood, brain tissue, nerve fibers, milk, yolk of egg, and
     in the liver, kidneys, and adrenal glands. It constitutes a large
     part of most gallstones and occurs in atheroma of the arteries.
chyrurgery: old English term for "surgery"
cilia: tiny hairlike structures attached to certain cells to protect them
     from injury
cirrhosis: a disease in which there is hardening of an organ, particularly
     of the liver
clinical: related to disease in patients
co-carcinogen: a substance that acts with a carcinogen to produce
     cancer

coronary: related to the coronary vessels that supply blood to the heart muscle

death certificate: a form that physicians are required to fill out concerning persons who have died

death rate: see *mortality rate*

diabetes: a disease due to a deficiency of insulin

DNA: deoxyribonucleic acid, a nucleoprotein which occurs in the chromosomes of cells and is responsible for their effects upon growth, reproduction, and other cellular processes and activities; occurs also in some viruses

duodenum: the first portion of the small intestine, connects with the stomach

electrocardiogram: a record of the electrical waves produced by the heartbeat

embolus: a piece of a blood clot or other material, such as a particle of fat, which is carried by the bloodstream and causes obstruction when it lodges in a blood vessel too small for it to pass through

emphysema: a chronic disease in which the lungs lose their elasticity and lung tissue is eventually destroyed

endocrine gland: a gland producing a chemical substance which passes directly into the bloodstream and affects various functions and organs

epidemiology: the science of the study of the conditions under which diseases occur

epidermoid: arising from or similar to the cells of covering tissues, such as the skin or mucous membranes

epinephrine: an internal secretion of the adrenal gland, also called adrenalin

esophagus: the portion of the digestive tract that connects the mouth with the stomach

etiology: cause

fluoresce: to glow under certain kinds of light
FCC: Federal Communications Commission
FTC: Federal Trade Commission

Galen: a distinguished Roman physician of the second century
genes: the basic elements which transmit hereditary characteristics and
    of which chromosomes are composed
genetic: related to or dependent upon genes
goiter: an enlargement of the thyroid gland

habituation: a tendency to do something frequently, usually on a psy-
    chological basis
hallucination: perception of objects which are not real
hemoglobin: a chemical compound in the red corpuscles which carries
    oxygen and gives blood its red color
hormone: a chemical substance produced in one organ and carried in
    the blood to another organ or part of the body where it stimu-
    lates functional activity
hydrocarbon: a chemical molecule containing carbon and hydrogen
hydrogen cyanide: a highly poisonous gas
hypnosis: an induced sleeplike condition in which the subject responds
    to the suggestion of the hypnotist

infarction, myocardial: an area of heart muscle that dies because its
    blood supply has been cut off
inhalation: breathing in; an inward breath
in situ: local; in one spot

larynx: the voice box
leukemia: a malignant (cancerous) disease of the white blood cells
leukoplakia: whitish spots or areas on the skin or the inside of the
    cheeks or the tongue; frequently precancerous
life expectancy: years an individual may be expected to live beyond a
    given age
lobeline: a chemical compound similar to nicotine

longevity: length of life
lumen: an opening

malignant: dangerous; tending to produce death
metastasis: the transfer of disease from one organ to another by means
of blood or lymph
mortality: death
mortality rate: the number of deaths in a given unit of the population,
usually the number per 100,000 persons
mortality ratio: the ratio of one mortality (or death) rate to another.
For example, if we consider the mortality rate of nonsmokers
as 1 and the mortality rate of pipe smokers as 20 percent
higher, the mortality ratio is 1.2; if the mortality rate of cigarette smokers is 2½ times as high as that of nonsmokers, the
mortality ratio is 2.5.

narcotic: a drug that relieves pain and induces sleep: in large doses it
causes stupor, coma, or even death
National Clearinghouse for Smoking and Health: a division of the
U.S. Public Health Service which collects and disseminates information on this health problem and promotes measures for
its control
nicotine: a highly toxic chemical that occurs in tobacco
nitrogen dioxide: one of the poisonous gases that occurs in cigarette
smoke

palpitation: rapid, forceful beating of the heart
pancreas: an important gland, in the upper part of the abdomen, that
secretes digestive juices and insulin
pathologist: a physician who specializes in the examination of diseased
tissues
pathology: the branch of medicine that deals with disease processes
peptic ulcer: ulcer of stomach or duodenum
peripheral vascular disease: disease of the blood vessels, particularly of
the extremities: arms, legs, hands, and feet
phenol: a chemical also called "carbolic acid"

physick: old English term for "medical treatment"
plaques: smooth, flat areas on the skin or mucous membranes
precancerous: preceding cancer
predispose: make more susceptible
prospective: forward-looking
Public Health Service: the major agencies of the United States government concerned with health

retrospective: looking backward in time
RNA: ribonucleic acid, a chemical substance that acts as an intermediary between DNA and the cytoplasm of the cell, thought to be associated with protein synthesis; occurs also in some viruses

scurvy: a deficiency disease due to lack of vitamin C
sinusitis: inflammation of the paranasal sinuses
snuff: powdered tobacco
spasm: a sudden, involuntary muscular contraction
statistics: numerical facts assembled and classified so as to present significant information
stroke: a sudden paralysis, usually with partial or complete loss of consciousness and sensation; caused by interference with circulation to the brain
Surgeon General: the chief executive officer of the U.S. Public Health Service

tar (tobacco): a brown sticky mass, condensed from tobacco smoke, that contains nicotine and a number of carcinogenic chemicals
thalidamide: a sleep-inducing drug which, when taken by pregnant women, caused some deformities of offspring
therapy: treatment
thorax: the chest
thrombus: a clot which forms on the inside of a blood vessel
toxic: poisonous
tumor: an abnormal mass in the body; it may or may not be dangerous to health

ulcer: an open sore other than a wound

ultraviolet light: invisible short rays in sunlight, beyond the violet end
of the spectrum (rainbow). These rays are irritating, cause
tanning of the skin, and change certain oils in the skin to
vitamin D.

virus: exceedingly small forms of living material that cause certain
diseases. Varying in size and shape, they cannot be seen with
an ordinary microscope but can be studied with electron mi-
croscopes which magnify up to a million times.

INDEX